Mark Stewart-Jones was born in London and brought up in South Wales. He has worked variously as a writer, musician, life model, Tarot card reader and rare-book dealer. Today he lives with his partner and his daughter, Sophie, dividing his time between Canterbury and Paris. He has had three novels published by Book Guild Publishing: *Martin Bonehouse* (1996), *An Ecstasy of Fumbling* (1998) and *Every Other Inch a Gentleman* (2007).

By the same author:

Martin Bonehouse, The Book Guild, 1996
An Ecstasy of Fumbling, The Book Guild, 1998
Every Other Inch a Gentleman, The Book Guild, 2007

DAUGHTER

Mark Stewart-Jones

Illustrations by Sophie Stewart-Jones

Book Guild Publishing
Sussex, England

First published in Great Britain in 2009 by
The Book Guild
Pavilion View
19 New Road
Brighton, East Sussex
BN1 1UF

Typesetting in Goudy by
Keyboard Services, Luton, Bedfordshire

Printed in Great Britain by
Athenaeum Press Ltd, Gateshead

A catalogue record for this book is available from
The British Library

ISBN 978 1 84624 293 9

For anyone who ever had a little faith

Contents

First Season

Good Days and Bad Days

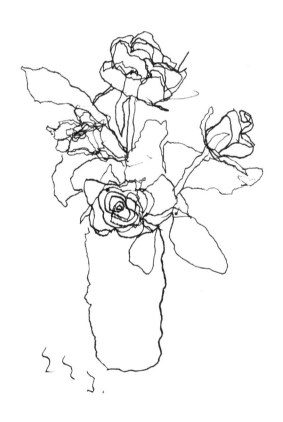

You are three hours old when I hear someone use the word 'she' for the very first time.

Referring directly to you, the use of the word takes me completely by surprise and I realise that right up until this moment you have been lacking any suggestion of specific gender or identity. You have simply been the epicentre of crisis and panic. You exist only within the confines of 'a very serious problem' or solely in relation to 'the complications'.

These complications have left you tiny and scared and struggling for your life, barely visible through tubes and turmoil and monitors. Through the panels of the incubator, you look pale and exhausted but still you are fighting. Meanwhile, the doctor is explaining to me that you have suffered a 'tremendous shock to the brain during delivery' and I nod automatically at this.

He continues talking. But *diagnosis, prognosis, care, assessment* all seem concepts belonging to a different place and time altogether. Instead I am witnessing some primal human drama, the most basic struggle for life.

I explain to him vaguely that your mother is back on the maternity ward recovering from her ordeal and I have been sent down to see how you are doing. I speak as though I have no notion of the severity of the situation. But this is not a true reflection of my state of mind. By this point, everything that I once understood to be me has been shattered and reassembled and divided into two, a new duality, parallel, consecutive. The internal, what I am feeling and the external, what I see taking place in front of me. They are at once a product of one another but somehow distinct and unrelated. I try and imagine what you must be going through even for a moment but it's a futile conceit.

The doctor mentions the foetal distress during labour and the lack of oxygen during the final stages of the delivery. Then he concludes by saying that 'she will have to be monitored very closely now'.

The shock of hearing this word passes and I begin to take great comfort from it. I root myself firmly in the moment and I feel that my presence at your side is suddenly not simply justified but actually required. I feel less like a spectator, less helpless, less useless.

From this word another two extrapolate themselves and in an instant, there is something else: a fleeting spark of certainty. Something very precious on to which I can hold while all about me takes on the stasis of nightmare.

Whatever happens now, beyond these moments, whatever is lost, whatever may have been denied us, there are the two words that I will not let anyone take away from us. Ever.

Father.

Daughter.

You are two days old when I get a phone call at 7.30 in the morning informing me that you have taken a turn for the worse. I wake your mother, who discharged herself from the hospital the previous evening, and we rush to see you.

You have been, for the past 36 hours, in the Special Care Baby Unit (referred to by the hospital staff rather awkwardly as SCBU or phonetically 'scaboo'; it is an Intensive Care ward for babies, low birth weight, premature or, like you, those with 'problems'.) It is a ward or more accurately a room with six or so incubators and a bewildering array of equipment. You are still in your incubator and hooked up to a ventilator, which has been assisting your breathing. It has been explained to us by the consultant that the doctor on duty 'mismanaged' the latter stages of the delivery. While his tone remained conciliatory and sympathetic to an extent, he made very few direct references

4

to your condition. But I have been able to stroke your hand a couple of times while I sit and talk to you and this has been our first tangible contact. At one point in the afternoon you opened your eyes and looked at me. It was obviously a greater thrill for me as you immediately went back to sleep.

We arrive at the ward about eight o'clock and somebody tells me, it might have been a doctor, it might have been a nurse (in crises you recall information, not necessarily the source) that there are problems with your lungs – you have also started to have fits.

'I am afraid,' the same voice tells me, 'that she might be slipping away now.'

This has been the great underlying, unspoken fear of the past two days. I realise that as parents we have been living minute-by-minute and hour-by-hour, daring to look no further than the immediate. The news is the unbolting of a door and suddenly I feel numb, the same numbness I recall from other accounts of people in the midst of personal tragedy. I once assumed that this was about having no feelings, no connection, that the brain was blocking things out as a survival impulse. But I'm older now. It's not a question of feeling nothing, it is more that the person feels *everything* simultaneously, every conceivable emotion in the range of human experience, all forced through a single flashing instant so it is impossible to identify a single dominant sensation.

I nod vaguely at this but find myself suddenly overwhelmed by the strongest impulse. It becomes stronger and stronger and I have to restrain myself.

Now, I think, now is the time!

Just watch me!

I am going to push my way through doctors and nurses and hurl myself towards your incubator. Before they even know what I am doing I will pick you up, wrestle you free of tubes and wires and sensors and run out of the hospital with you. If you have only a day, an hour, a minute, I tell myself, then let it be with someone who loves you. In two days you have known nothing aside from pain and fear. Know what it is like to feel loved and cherished if only for the tiniest fraction of time. (Proportionally speaking, if a child only has a lifespan of a couple of days then an hour or so is surely a significant time!) I will hold you; let you feel the warmth of another human being, to know company and humanity.

They will try and stop us but we will be too quick for them. We will run and run, far away from here and now. It will be just the two of us. We will have adventures, we will prove them wrong – we will prove them *all* wrong! I will keep you close to me always; if the last thing you ever see is my face then at least it will be the face of someone who loves you.

Meanwhile someone is saying something about a final blessing.

'A what?' I ask blankly.

'You know, a final blessing, the hospital chaplain will come and do it. It's very quick. A nice service though. He's nice too, you'll like him.'

I realise what I am being told and again I nod silently.

I think to myself that at least they will let one of us hold you during your blessing. But I am not thinking it, I realise that I am actually saying it. Your mother and I talk it over and agree that I should be the one to have you on my lap. I tell the staff this but rather than generate the positive response I would have anticipated, my request achieves precisely the opposite effect. This, the combined wisdom of a doctor and three nurses insists, is not at all a good idea.

'What,' they ask, 'if *something* happens?' How would I cope? I explain that I am quite aware of this but don't regard it as a consideration. I say that I want my daughter to feel loved even if it is only for a short time but I know that they have stopped listening. While they still consider my request a monumentally bad idea they eventually accede.

The chaplain arrives and looks reassuringly ecclesiastical. He exudes wisdom and kindness.

He looks at me and smiles. I smile back. For some reason I remember the story of another chaplain, this one was actually the vicar who performed the wedding ceremony for my parents in 1953. In his earlier years he too had been a chaplain and during the Great War he was active overseas. Amongst his duties, he had actually given the last rites to Rupert Brooke.

Another chaplain.

Another blessing.

Then, without warning, for the first time in two days, I miss my mum and dad.

They would know what to do.

The chaplain introduces himself and I feel acutely sorry for him. Of all the duties he must be called upon to perform, this surely must be the most painful. We are all aware that this is a place where his God is so often questioned and accused.

He asks me your name and I say that it's Sophie.

I am shown where to sit and after much manoeuvring and negotiating with tubes, wires and sensors (a process that requires the assistance of two nurses) you are finally placed on my lap. The profound sense of joy I experience is such that I am hardly aware of the service. You open your eye at one point and we look at each other. I feel that I have kept a promise and, whatever nameless thing that passes between us at this moment, it will live with me for the rest of my life.

I recall nothing of the blessing and when it is over and a nurse comes to take you from me I am once again gripped with the desire to hold you and rush for the exits. Common sense or cowardice prevails and you are returned to your incubator.

In the afternoon your mother and I have a long chat with the paediatrician who comes to see you. He explains to us at length the true extent of the 'problem' and what the term 'brain damage' actually means when applied to newborn babies. It is not a particularly heartening speech. However, he doesn't shy away from discussing the very real threat that is facing you at the moment: the functioning of the lungs. In basic terms, you are not breathing well enough on your own and if you don't start breathing unassisted very soon then this ventilator becomes effectively a life-support system.

Your brain suffered a 'tremendous insult' during birth and 'the next twenty-four hours will be critical' and he prepares us that we might face some difficult decisions.

As the afternoon progresses, your breathing becomes shallower and shallower and at five o' clock we find ourselves presented with that difficult decision. You are no longer breathing on your own and, solemnly, we are told by the paediatrician that we must decide if we want you to remain on the ventilator indefinitely, knowing that this is the only thing keeping you alive, or do we simply allow 'nature to take its course'.

Suddenly you and I are running again through forests and across deserts knowing that we can never stop. It might be minutes now or even seconds but something of us will live for ever. If you can't walk I will carry you, if you can't talk then we will find another way.

'Do you think we can have some time to think about this?' I ask mechanically.

The paediatrician makes a face and looks at his watch. 'Well, I can give you about ... half an hour. Sorry.'

Your mother and I stumble out of the hospital into the bright afternoon sun. Buildings, roads, pavements, people, cars swim around me and never in my life have I felt so exiled from the physical world.

Half an hour?

Your mother and I look at each other and feel helpless, we share the source of our pain perhaps but we can't share the pain. Her pain is a mother's pain and more focused than mine. She's angry too, angry at everyone. But I can't ease her agonies any more than she can ease mine. The sudden rush of isolation is unbearable.

In five hours I have experienced all the joy, the love, the

hope, the despair, the anguish and anxiety that it takes most fathers years to experience.

You managed to achieve this in a few hours!

Now I can approach your situation as a mature adult.

I hear myself calmly saying that the fairest approach would be to let you decide. It must be your decision, not that of your parents or some doctor. You must be granted that level of dignity and your wishes must be respected, whatever they may be.

I feel uncomfortable at the prospect of keeping you alive against your will simply because I would be unable to deal with the loss.

We return to SCBU and inform the staff there of our decision. In our absence, however, they have been trying a different combination of drugs to control the fits. It appears that the original medication was sedating you so effectively that it was causing your breathing to become shallow. You are a much better colour than before and sleeping soundly.

'It's only the first hurdle of many,' a nurse remarks, probably imagining that she is doing the kindest thing.

I ignore her and gaze through the glass of the incubator.

'Rest now, daughter,' I whisper. 'You've had a busy day, you must be exhausted...'

You are eleven years and 95 days old and we are back in hospital again. The diagnosis has certain miserable implications and I receive the news as stoically as possible. It would be an understatement to say that I was anticipating this particular outcome and as I'm invited by the doctor to review the X-rays the procedure qualifies simply as confirmation.

A butterfly fracture in your left femur.

You have broken your leg.

Not that, in fairness, you played an active part in its fracture, you are just the unwilling, unfortunate recipient of wretched misfortune and circumstance. An accident, pure and simple, a terrible, stupid, avoidable accident. A completely freak occurrence they are saying. Not that there is the slightest comfort to be gleaned from this conclusion.

I go over the incident with the doctor and he explains that due to your increased muscle tone and the stiffness in your legs in combination with what he sensitively terms their 'under-use' you are vulnerable to this sort of rupture. While you were lying on your back, following your bath, it seems the simple act of moving your leg and twisting it slightly in a particular way resulted in the fracture. I am just about to point out that I am not actually the person responsible for this but stop myself just in time as I realise that I'm listening to a diagnosis and not a direct accusation.

Now comes the news I have been dreading. We are to remain for at least six weeks in hospital now while your leg is in traction healing. In short we will spend the rest of the summer in hospital. It seems such a cruel twist (of both fate and leg) that we were about to set off for Venice for a few days to celebrate my birthday and instead we find ourselves marooned in Sidcup General.

So, these must be just the tears of bitter irony, I tell myself.

You have been given a massive dose of painkillers and are fairly subdued when we are taken up to the ward and shown into a side room adjacent to the main reception area. This is going to be our new home, I tell you, but you seem unimpressed and I don't blame you.

By this point, your leg has been put in plaster and very shortly we are introduced to the whole apparatus of traction. It is an aspect of medicine of which, up until this moment, I have been wholly ignorant and I confess that in the 21st century, in an epoch of laser surgery and cloning, the underlying principle and resulting mechanisms do strike an oddly medieval note. But I am just going to have to get used to it.

You look so tiny in your hospital bed and gown and I am sure I detect a slight sadness in your eyes. This is a rare

10

occurrence in a young lady so ceaselessly positive and optimistic. Sometimes, I suppose, all this bravery must be a bit exhausting.

I am given a mattress, which means I'll be able to sleep on the floor next to your bed. Then should you need anything in the night I'll be right next to you. Meanwhile, abandoning myself to our situation, I boldly conclude that if this room is going to be our home for the next month or so I should attempt to make it a little more homely for us. So, with this end in mind, I gather up some necessary items from the house and drag them in. Portable CD player, laptop etc. Thus we now find ourselves in familiar unfamiliar surroundings – a Spartan and greatly edited version of our own lives. The *Reader's Digest* adaptation. For some reason, I assume this is what it must be like staying in a caravan. But I don't want to think about that. It reminds me of holidays.

Everyone has now gone to Venice as planned and the two of us are completely alone. It takes me a while to appreciate the significance of this. But over the following couple of days it slowly occurs to me that we are actually more alone than we've been in a long time.

Just the two of us again.

Officially too, as I have now been a single parent for almost two years.

Within a day or so of our arrival, a routine is firmly established. A nurse will pop in a couple of times a day and check your temperature, every so often a doctor will examine your leg and check the weights, and at least once a day someone will tell me I look tired but that's about it. The rest of the time we are largely left to our own devices. The days are long, interminable and featureless. They lack any kind of light and shade and it is not long before I am amusing myself by recognising in my behaviour the slow but definite process of institutionalisation. I catch myself delighting in the prospect of meal times but only for the way they satisfyingly divide the day into less eternal fractions.

I try to keep you entertained and stimulated as best I can but it is not easy, you are still very drowsy from the painkillers and I'm told the best thing for you is to sleep as much as you can.

So I watch you sleep.

You are eleven years and 97 days old and we share a birthday I am unlikely to forget in a while. The day is marked by a quick trip downstairs to the canteen to buy a muffin. This I divide in two and I sing very quietly to you:

Happy birthday to me...
Happy birthday to me...

This, I must confess, is a unique moment in my experience of birthday celebrations. It is also a fairly bleak one and perhaps as a consequence neither of us seems that interested in the muffin.

Happy birth...

Hospitals!
You've had a couple of spells in hospital over the years but our visits have never been beyond a few weeks. This will be by far our longest stay and today at some vague, nameless point between afternoon tea and supper I have one of those hospital moments with you again. I do try and avoid these things. I attempt to place all manner of obstacles in the way but resistance is hopeless. It happens every time and, with diminishing conviction, I usually ascribe it to tiredness, dehydration or bad diet. This afternoon, without any build-up or warning, as I am giving you your drink I am suddenly overwhelmed by that familiar and most profound of all sensations. Not happy or sad. Beyond anything I could denote simply as

good or bad. I think I can best describe it as a fleeting epiphany, what is called a *satori* in Zen Buddhism. A moment of complete awareness. Its effects may linger indefinitely but the initial spark flares only for a moment. It happens whenever the barricades of distraction fail me and I'm inadvertently forced to recall your first few weeks of life.

(A long time ago – but forever passing and never completely passed.)

This is a reconnection as much as a recollection and it only happens under these precise conditions. A time whenever the word *helpless* applies equally to both of us. A time rather like now. I look into your eyes and remember everything, the word, line and chapter of all our days, as it is all compressed and distilled into a single heartbeat. I travel back and forward in the fraction of an instant and experience every joy and every agony, every moment of love and pain in the blinking of an eye. It is something that resonates in me as our point of departure and reminds me of who I am and sometimes maybe I need to be reminded of it.

And talking of pain.

Today is also the day that the doctors decide to reduce the level of your painkillers. They explain that this may cause a few problems but it's not good for you to be on such high doses for more than a couple of days. I am told that you may find the transition a bit difficult.

At around your bedtime this becomes all too apparent, you are crying and distressed and obviously in a great deal of pain. Nurses pop their heads around our door from time to time and chuck me the odd sympathetic smile but they can do very little else to help you. I ask if there's anything at all I can give you but they remind me that you are not due anything until the morning. I start trying to explain that usually you have an amazingly high pain threshold, *no, really an amazingly high threshold*, and you've coped and dealt with so much pain in the past, *more pain than most of us would endure in silence*, and it would take a great deal to make you this upset and you are obviously in some pretty major discomfort. *So, if there's any chance . . .*

But there isn't any chance and the doctor will be around in the morning in what I calculate to be roughly ten hours' time. It is going to be a long night. Your crying gets louder and having run through all the usual pacifiers, I push the chair next to the bed and rest my head near yours so we are looking directly at each other. Maybe it was my *satori* earlier but, struggling to make myself heard over the sound of your crying and approaching the point of desperation, I devise a new game to play with you. It is possibly infantile and ill conceived but it's all I have.

I talk softly to you as though we are sharing a great confidence and remind you of how much we have shared together in eleven years, all the adventures we've had together, all the problems we've taken on together. Together. It's when we're at our best, I tell you. As you pointed out a long time ago, we understand each other and we're a good team. If we had nothing else going for us that would still be enough for me. Your crying intensifies but by this time the idea has crystallized in my head and I continue. We are not doing this together, I tell you, we are not sharing any of this, I'm so sorry, Sophie, but I can't help you with your pain because I don't understand it. I have no idea what you are feeling. This is something that you are going through on your own.

Of course, I might be able to help if I could just feel some of your agony. If you could just share some of it with me. I lean over so my forehead is almost touching yours. I tell you that you must really concentrate, harder than you've ever concentrated before, you must really try and focus your mind for a moment and just do this one thing for me. I need you to think really hard and send some of your pain to me. Then I can know what you are feeling and then we can share it. You won't have so much pain to deal with if we divide it between us. That's obvious isn't it? Come on, Sophie, concentrate really

14

hard. I have to as well. Come on. No. That didn't work, I'm not getting anything. You need to really give this everything, try again. I say nothing for a few moments. No, sorry still nothing... Ow! No, wait a minute I felt something then, ouch, that was really painful. And again! No wonder you've been so upset, this is horrible isn't it? Keep sending it to me, Sophie, you must keep concentrating... Ow! That was a bad one, well done...

This game continues roughly in this fashion for about ten minutes. I confess I have absolutely no idea what I'm actually doing and I have never attempted anything like this in the past. But I urge you to concentrate and remind you that the more you give your pain to me the more it should begin to ease.

Then I notice that you have stopped crying. Your eyes are closing and your body is relaxing. I am astonished by this and creep quietly away. I would have been tempted to speculate that you had just cried yourself to sleep and the timing of the game was coincidental. However, when you disturb a couple of hours later and I play the same game with you the results are the same.

During this second incident, I am subsequently informed, I am observed by a couple of nurses. The following morning they ask me about it and enquire if I have been taught cognitive visualisation techniques. I reply that I have no idea what they're talking about. Instead, I remind them of a scene at the end of the first Indiana Jones film. Harrison Ford is unveiling a fairly detailed plan and allocating various roles. Someone then asks him what he is going to do and he replies that he's just making it up as he goes along. That, I confess, is still pretty much my take on fatherhood.

Basically, I say, I'm just jamming.

You look tired, one of them says.

You are eleven years and 102 days old and we reach the end

15

of your first week in traction and our first week in Sidcup General.

Venice is particularly warm in August, I'm told and the beach at the Lido is fabulous.

Meanwhile, I take far greater delight in the news that your pain seems to have been brought under some control. Largely, I am sure, this is a result of the right cocktail of analgesics but I like to think that playing our little game helps a bit too. One of my main concerns at the moment is keeping you entertained and occupied while you're effectively bed-ridden for the next six weeks. This is something I would imagine to be a problem with any child, able-bodied or otherwise, but I do feel I should be chalking the days off on a wall somewhere.

It's hard for you to write at the moment, which is your usual and preferred method of communication, so we are forced to restrict ourselves to absolute essentials. Rather than let this encroach too much on our usual level of contact, I read to you a lot and we listen to music and all around us the days just go on and on and on...

In the evening I devise a variation on our game to help you sleep. From where you are lying in your fixed position our window looks out on to the trees at the rear of the hospital. I ask you to pretend that you are looking out of the window of a ship. For so many years now you have had this particular love of boats and the sea in general. Whenever we go anywhere you will always insist on the boat trip and have remarked in the past with your usual easy profundity that you are more yourself near water. So, looking out of our ship's window, you can guide us wherever in the world you would like us to go.

Faced with no real alternative during these conversations I am entirely reliant on upon what was probably your earliest and most primitive communication skill – your deliberate blinked response to indicate YES. I give you the various options as we go along and you make the choices for us by indicating in the affirmative.

Together, we gaze out at the limitless horizon and infinite possibility as I run through all the places from our past that you may wish to revisit. You are not interested in going to Memphis, Greenwich, Dublin, your Grandma's house or school. I'm slightly surprised to discover that you have no urge to travel back home either. No, you are absolutely determined that we sail your hospital boat to Paris! OK. I tell you to close your eyes and prepare yourself for the journey. We will not even think about lifting our anchor unless your eyes are shut tight.

Then, eschewing the remotest notion of geographical accuracy – naturally, I respect your intelligence but you are still only eleven and it's a magic boat anyway – I describe our journey. I tell you about all the places and the landmarks we pass on the way. I go into some detail about locations that are particularly familiar to you and remind you of various incidents in the past. We sail up the Seine and our trip naturally includes visits to the major tourist attractions like the Louvre and the Eiffel Tower but also we call at the little café off Rue de Rivoli, where the owner was so nice to us and so helpful that time, do you remember? He moved all the tables and chairs for us, it was lunchtime too. And that great children's clothes shop in St-Germain-des-Prés, where we had to go in a great hurry and buy you a raincoat because we'd got caught in a sudden downpour. Then there was that time we ...

But once again you have drifted off into a deep sleep.

As quietly and gently as possible, I kiss you on the forehead.

The end of another day.

Fatigue once again overwhelms me.

Good days and bad days.

I loathe that expression and the ease with which it slips off the tongue sometimes. It's usually trotted out as a stock answer and it discourages further enquiries but it only hints at the extremes and the scope of our lives together. A hundred rooms, a hundred faces and a hundred variations on the same questions.

Good days and bad days.

17

Many years ago as a rather desperate coping strategy, I devised a method of converting the word *normal* (without doubt one of the most loaded and variable words in regular use) into the word *ordinary*. Simple really, sleight of hand, another little game possibly, but to me it was an effective way of approaching the whole situation from a different angle. If I had to accept that you would never be *normal* in the narrow conventional sense then why allow *normal* to be the desired state? Who would crave the dullness and mediocrity of *ordinary*? Everyday we must strive to transcend such dreary restrictions and let us every day celebrate not your lack of *normality*, instead let us delight in the fact that you are truly *extraordinary*. You always have been and you always will be. As a direct and happy consequence of this, your life is lived on your terms. A rare gift and one that possibly implies a certain degree of intent and organisation on my part. This would have been a wonderfully noble deed but sadly I suspect that it is just another serendipitous by-product of the usual jamming.

Good days and bad days.

Yet this simple division does hint at the paradox that remains fairly central in my life with you. The eternal contradiction. It is something I accept and accommodate but not something I can easily explain. I can speak of the pain I have experienced, the great sadness, the endless anxieties and frustrations, the sleepless nights at the end of endless days and the overwhelming sense of total isolation, but these are nothing compared to the utter joy that fills my life every single moment I spend in your company.

I am so grateful that you have chosen to spend your life with me.

My daughter.

You are six days old and I get the briefest indication of some of the problems that lie ahead for us. It is an exchange that hindsight urges me to invest with an ominous resonance; the conversational equivalent of a couple of Van Gogh's black crows.

It occurs the morning that they attempt to take you off the ventilator. This proves to have been a rather hasty judgement and you are not breathing sufficiently well on your own to allow this to happen. You have been having fits too and the drugs that control the fits also affect your breathing. So, it's a very delicate balance.

A series of precarious moments.

The doctors are still reticent to get into many discussions about your prognosis but occasionally I find a degree of solace and comfort in a phrase I might hear like 'long-term situation' or 'future problems'. I have been reminded almost hourly for a whole week that the shock that you had to your brain during delivery and the resulting damage remains the most immediate problem.

They speak in terms of recovery but no one is under any illusions that the real issue is simply one of survival.

You've picked up a lung infection overnight and while this is considered a less serious condition and often results from being on a ventilator, when I come in to see you I am unable to take you out of your incubator. I'm a bit disappointed by this but I pull up a chair and sit next to you.

I am aware at this point that one of the doctors with whom I have just been discussing the anti-convulsants and breathing situation is standing behind me. Presuming he has nothing further to add I just disregard his presence. I'm quite content and oblivious, just chatting away to you and I notice that the corners of your mouth are moving.

I sense the doctor moving closer.

'That's nice,' he says. 'You can see that she recognises your voice.'

'Yes,' I say absently. But never being one to ignore the chance of provoking a positive word, I add, 'maybe that's an encouraging sign?'

He looks a little dubious. 'Is it?'

'Well,' I say cautiously. 'Doesn't that imply that her brain might not be as damaged as it's been suggested.'

'Why do you say that?'

'If she recognises my voice, that involves memory, doesn't it? Wouldn't that be a very positive thing?'

My evident naivety is conspicuously the source of some amusement to him and he smiles to himself.

'No,' he says, shaking his head. 'I'm afraid it isn't that simple. What we are witnessing here is instinct, not memory, I fear.'

I feel suitably chastised. 'So, recognition of a voice or anything for that matter is, in simple medical terms, an instinct?'

'In most cases.' He smiles again and evidently keen not to prolong the conversation any further he wanders off.

I do appreciate the accepted wisdom that states clearly that false hope is a deeply undesirable emotion. (Although, I suppose, this could be countered by suggesting that any hope, whether false or not, can be used in a positive way. Am I an optimist or simply a man in denial?) I do understand the caution and can usually see the reasoning but this conversation remains with me for a long time. It makes no logical sense to me whatsoever.

Either that or I still have a very great deal to learn.

I regain some composure in the afternoon and take great delight in referring to you and I as 'we', which is, I think, the first time that I have ever done this.

You are twelve days old and I discover something about myself I would rather not and our vocabulary is extended in a particular direction, irrevocably and permanently.

You are currently requiring the ventilator less and less and there is now talk of moving you out of the incubator and into a cot. I talk to the paediatrician this morning and notice a certain shift in his attitude towards you and the situation in general. He comments on how you have fought so hard and while we still have a long, long way to go he points out that this is an encouraging sign.

Technology and medicine can only go so far, he tells me, no one has yet devised a means of replicating or encouraging the will to live. That exists only within the individual and it is present (or not present) from the second we are born. He imparts this information with some confidence but I'm not convinced that we are still strictly in the realm of hardcore medical fact. For a moment we seem to be teetering on the brink of matters infinitely more abstract and metaphysical.

However, I must admit, the whole conversation does lift the spirits considerably. His approach is so different from that of some of the other staff I have encountered over the past week or so. Their general tone is usually one of caution, of not wishing to commit, of not wanting to encourage the dreaded false hope. When opinions are so divided it's difficult not to similarly divide the people who hold those opinions.

I talk to you about this while I have you on my lap a little later in the day. Your mother still finds herself unable to do this – no explanation is offered and I feel disinclined to question her on the subject. I tell you what the paediatrician said and slowly I begin my confession. It is one of the most deplorable and essentially pointless of all human characteristics and one I find as depressing in myself as I do in others. I try to stop myself but it is never easy. Not satisfied with simply agreeing or disagreeing with people, I still sometimes find myself subtly dividing up the population into 'Us' and 'Them'. As I have been doing with all the staff involved with you. It's a dismal trait and one that probably suggests a gross immaturity.

As this procedure possibly results from the most basic insecurities, I might even be tempted to consider forgiveness but I shouldn't be so easy on myself! With very little effort you could detect this particular method of thinking behind all manner of bigotry, prejudice and intolerance. I tell you that you mustn't grow up and think like this – it's really not good.

Towards the end of the afternoon, the doctor with whom I had the recognition/instinct conversation asks to speak to me. For a second it actually crosses my mind that he might have researched our discussion a little further and wants to share it with me. I couldn't be more wrong. He asks how you are and I say that you're doing a bit better today.

He doesn't reply to this, instead he continues in calm, measured tones, 'You've probably spoken to a lot of doctors recently, haven't you?'

'I suppose so.'

'Well, I was wondering, has anyone said ... I mean, have you heard the expression spasticity at all?'

'No,' I say.

'OK. Has anyone said anything about a brain scan?'

'I don't think so.'

'Right then, has anyone talked to you about cerebral palsy...?'

It is at this precise moment that these two words first enter our lives and there they will remain.

Having replied in the negative the doctor then concludes our conversation and I'm left to ponder its significance. Later in the evening, your mother goes home and I promise to follow on shortly after I've said goodbye to you properly. I make my way back up to the ward and find that the SCBU is dark and quiet. So, I creep stealthily up to your incubator and start whispering my goodnights to you.

Suddenly, behind me, there is a voice in the darkness. 'Do you believe in God?'

I turn around. 'Pard...?'

The question is repeated, modified by an additional emphasis. 'Do you *believe* in God?'

It is a woman's voice, strong, sonorous yet soothing; the voice of every mother in the whole world. 'I can hear you praying,' she says.

'No, I was just...'

I peer into the darkness and sitting behind me in the shadows is a nurse. I have no idea how long she has been sitting there and for a second or two I confess I feel acutely embarrassed. She tells me her name and smiles warmly at me.

At this precise moment, I feel like it is the first time in my life that someone has actually smiled at me.

'So, tell me,' she continues, 'do you believe in God?'

'Er ... well ... yes, probably, I suppose so,' I say awkwardly, presuming the question to be slanted somewhat.

'You see, Sophie is not supposed to die, God knows that. He will not let her die.'

I have absolutely no idea what to say in response to this so I simply smile and thank her. Then she asks me if you have any brothers or sisters and I reply in the negative.

I glance through the panels of the incubator at you and then back towards the nurse. I am half expecting no one to be there, just an empty chair and the vague scent of meadows and summers and flowers in the air.

I am reassured to find her in the process of getting up and wandering off in search of a cup of tea.

The whole conversation has an oddly ethereal, otherworldly quality and despite my earlier confession, the overwhelming desire to divide people into Us and Them sadly seems as resilient as it ever was.

You are eighteen days old and there is some encouraging news. When I arrive at the hospital this morning I find that you have been moved into a cot! The level of sedation has been decreased and you are now awake for long periods.

I feel overjoyed and my good mood lasts all morning until I see the paediatrician. He tells me that your breathing is still a little erratic and he's concerned that it might not be entirely a result of the chest infection. You are still having fits periodically and he warns me that there is the possibility that its cause is the massive damage to the brain stem. This might in addition affect your capacity to feed, which is why it is so important that you start taking some milk, otherwise there will be even more impossible decisions.

The next 48 hours will be critical, by which he means of course that they will be *even more* critical.

The next day I manage to get you to take a tiny bit of milk. Not enough to warrant a major celebration but certainly no one would deny that it is a nod in the right direction. Yet I remain concerned that even though you have been off the ventilator for a little while now, you still haven't been able to cry.

Now your eyes are open there are moments when you stare at me.

Blankly.

Vacantly.

Absently.

And I am terrified.

I forget who I am, where I am and everything that has ever happened to me. I just recall something about massive damage to the brain stem. A panic passes over me and I discover that, like the opposite of love is not hate, the opposite of hope is not fear.

The opposite of both is doubt.

Later in the day this mood lifts somewhat when I have a brief chat with the nurse from the other night. I have seen her a couple of times these past few days but since our first encounter this was the first time we'd exchanged anything beyond a smile or the briefest hello. I am walking down the corridor back towards the SCBU, after buying a drink from the machine, when I see her coming in the opposite direction.

'How are you?' she asks.

'I'm fine,' I say without thinking.

She smiles and fixes me with a stare. 'It's all about faith, you know. You must always have faith. You must believe that.'

'Faith in Sophie, you mean?'

'Of course.'

'I have every faith in Sophie.'

She touches my arm. 'Sometimes faith can be even more important than love, and this is all about faith, you must never forget that.'

She says goodbye and I watch her disappearing from view down the escalator and suddenly I feel totally alone. I repeat her words to myself as I make my way back to the SCBU.

This is all about faith.

You are three weeks and 2 days old and I manage to get you to drink 25 ml of milk. The target is 60 ml so we are nearly half way there. But our day is overshadowed by the news that the tiny premature baby, who had been in the incubator next to your cot, died last night.

His name was Toby and I see his parents this morning when they come into the SCBU to collect his bits and pieces. I feel sick and can only make fleeting eye contact. We've shared one another's crises for almost a month but that has to end now. I want to say something but whenever you really need the power of language, it deserts you.

There are no words for this.

There is only something momentarily glimpsed behind the eyes.

Toby was born at 30 weeks and had fought against overwhelming odds to get as far as he did.

'How's Sophie this morning?' Toby's mother asks me as she is leaving and the look of pain on her face is unbearable.

Later on a nurse tells me, as if imparting a great confidence, that little girls in SCBU 'usually do better' than little boys.

Walking back home from the hospital at dusk tonight, I pass

some children playing football in the street and I think of three things. Totally unrelated but today somehow there seems to be this elaborate connection.

Firstly, I remember playing football as a kid during that vague, murky period in my development (those dark ages identified as being somewhere between Manchester United's European Cup win against Benfica and 'Ride A White Swan'). A handful of us would play after school on the common, staying on and on until it started to get dark. One boy would go home for his tea, then another couple would drift away and so on. Yet there was always the one who was left, the one who remained, carrying on kicking that ball around long after it was feasible to do so.

The one that refused to acknowledge the darkness.

A couple of times it might have even been me but usually it was a fat boy called Colin. Colin would insist he could see the ball perfectly well and that we must have all been blind or something. The game wasn't over as far as Colin was concerned – the game was never over. We would drift away and hear Colin's shouts in the darkness.

Alongside this image prompted obviously by the kids in the street, I thought about that passage in Céline's *Journey to the End of the Night*. He writes about how some fatally wounded soldiers would continue looting right up until their final breath, picking up things that might prove useful to them in the future. Not because they didn't realise they were dying but more because they didn't want something like a bullet in the head to spoil their day.

When some people die they have been doing so for decades, others do not even start dying until that very last moment.

I leave Céline and the footballers and my thoughts return to you and I think of you fighting and fighting and maybe even starting to make some progress now against all the odds. I think of 'long-term problems' but then I think of 'long-term' and of hope and possibility and of that simple refusal to acknowledge the darkness.

Then I think of little Toby.

And I don't think I will ever be able to put into words just how I feel tonight.

During the following couple of days the atmosphere in the SCBU is very different. Something can be perceived in the nurses's demeanour. I sense that there is a rediscovered purposefulness, a determination, as though it is all just a bit difficult at the moment and they are all having to concentrate that little bit harder.

Meanwhile you come very close to crying today.

You're not the only one.

You are four weeks old and I manage to get you to drink 60 ml! It probably doesn't sound like much of a landmark to anyone else but I feel we should be celebrating. You obviously share my excitement as at the conclusion you produce a couple of little contented squeaks. Your mother observes and offers encouragement although she still finds the whole situation distressing. She is still very angry too, angry about what is still euphemistically referred to as the 'mismanagement' of your birth. There is, I realise, a process that we are both going through at the moment. Being of a less independent cast, I realise that I am rather dependent upon you, my daughter, and I'm taking great comfort and inspiration from your strength and your bravery and your absolute refusal to give up.

I have a chat with you afterwards about something that's been playing on my mind recently. I suppose all parents, even those who would claim on their own behalf the most liberal of credentials, make plans for their children. Some would possibly claim to make unconscious plans and I feel that I fall into this category. Although, I suppose, if I'm honest, I was looking forward to one day introducing you to Raymond Chandler, The Marx Brothers, The Clash, Dylan Thomas, Big

Bill Broonzy, Jacques Tati, Thelonious Monk, *Thunderbirds* and I could make lists like this all day. Now, with the damage to your brain all that has gone, that version of our lives has been wiped away, stolen from us and you are a clean slate again. I have no idea what the future holds for you or for us – I can't even begin to guess. It's still debatable that you will ever leave hospital.

Apart from 60 ml of milk I have little or no influence and I realise you are your own person already. You are in charge here and you make your decisions.

If I am unable to picture you at the age of five, nine or thirteen or even imagine you next week, it is because I have no means of anticipating or influencing your decisions. This is something that I imagine all parents must endure ultimately – I am just going through the process a little sooner than most.

So, it becomes the absolute existential experience and I am rooted in every moment but only for the precise duration of that moment.

Desperate to conclude these deliberations on a positive note, I explain to you that if I am going to teach you things then it's only fair that the process should work both ways. I must learn to observe and understand. All I know at this time is that I just want the best for you. If there is the slightest flicker of a chance, a hope or a possibility, I want to be able to help you make the most of it.

I cannot conceive of doing anything more worthwhile with my life.

I want you to be able to capitalise on any potential that might be there. If I have to I will create a world for you and around you. I am tired and I sound stupid and over melodramatic but there is some truth in what I say to you.

And a promise.

It's a promise that will bring me into conflict with orthodox opinion and authority, with doctors and teachers and anybody else who knows you better than I do. It will be a struggle that will bring me to the brink of psychological and emotional exhaustion but if I could do it all over again, I would not change a single moment.

As I leave you I repeat the same half sung little mantra I have started singing to you every night:

If you can't walk, Daddy will carry you
If you can't talk, we'll just find another way...

You are five weeks and 3 days old when you leave the SCBU for the first time. We are taken by ambulance to another local hospital where you undergo a brain scan. This has been discussed at length recently and finally it is decided that an appointment should be made for the afternoon. I accompany you for the trip and at one point I am allowed to push you in a pram marked 'property of SCBU'. This is something in which I take particular delight. Moments of such divine normality have been denied us so often in this past month and a half that such a simple act can take on quite significant dimensions. You seem noticeably underwhelmed by the whole experience and sleep soundly throughout the whole visit.

On returning to the SCBU I have a chat with your paediatrician. I talk about the scan and he explains that it will be a day or two before the results are available. Cautiously then, he makes a reference to you leaving hospital. This is the first time he has done this and I try and get him to commit himself beyond 'at some point in the future'. Eventually I get a 'fairly soon' and finally 'in a couple of weeks maybe'. He adds that your mother and I have shown ourselves to be very able parents but I wasn't listening. I couldn't hear him above the sound of gently beating angels' wings and the choir of pink soprano cherubs that had just started bellowing in my ear in their perfect miniature harmony.

In a couple of weeks maybe...

I rejoin the conversation just as he is raising some concern about your fits and the necessity of getting them under control. From his tone I gather that he regards them as a challenge or a conundrum and not as anything life threatening. It seems it's a question of using the right combination of drugs. I rush to your cot and break the news to you.

'We're going home, daughter...' I whisper to you as you open a sleepy eye to look at me.

The following morning I sit and write my diary before I come to see you. I have no idea what precise vanity encourages a person to keep a diary. Surely it presupposes that a life is worth recording. That posterity requires its witness! In my defence, I weakly offer that I keep a diary only because I have always kept a diary. Yet, as I now discover, at times of crisis it can be a great means of focusing the mind. There is also a certain comfort in the continuity it provides.

I am not able to speak for myself but I do notice the change in your mother. Now as there seems to be an end in sight and we are less reliant on nervous energy, she looks totally exhausted. Everything you could recognise has been eroded or drilled out of her. I probably look no better.

Another meeting with the paediatrician during which the results of the CT brain scan are discussed. He points out the areas of damage to me but admits that there was less than he had expected. Although, he says, any prognosis regarding your development at this stage could be no more than speculative.

I ask rather bravely what areas in your life will be affected by the damage.

'Growth and learning,' he says.

This somewhat evasive answer puzzles me slightly as I suppose *growth and learning* covers pretty much the whole Being a Baby thing but before I can arrange these doubts into a sensible question he concludes by saying, 'We just have to wait and see.'

I nod my head and decide this is a sensible point to end our conversation.

You surviving the first three weeks of your life might be reasonably considered a miracle. Praying for two miracles in such a young life might well be considered unreasonable.

You are eleven years and 107 days old and with all necessary discretion I sneak away from the ward for a couple of hours this evening to allow your mother to visit you. Luckily our paths do not cross and she has left by the time I return. She visits once a week and I endeavour to avoid direct contact with her. There has remained a fairly constant level of bad feeling between she and I this past year. Sadly, this antipathy periodically manifests itself as fairly heated vocal confrontation and I feel that this is best avoided under the current circumstances. For your sake as much as mine.

So I cycle home and have a shower.

When I return you are alone again apart from the unfamiliar nurse who is giving your face and hands a wash. She informs me that your mother left about ten minutes ago and then she introduces herself, explaining that this is her first day back at work after returning from holiday. We chat for a little while and I trot out the usual potted biography. You are my only child and you have cerebral palsy, you can't walk, you have very little independent movement, you have no speech and are entirely reliant on others for all your care. Yet despite all this you are a bright, intelligent young person who communicates by writing and harbours ambitions to one day be an artist and live in Paris.

She smiles at this information in a manner that seems refreshingly free of condescension. She makes some passing reference to you being a daddy's girl and then, following quite evidently an earlier exchange with your mother, she asks me if I get to see you regularly.

I take a deep breath and with some reluctance I commence the optional appendix to the potted biography. I explain that you live with me and that I've always looked after you. In actual fact, it was always planned that I would stay at home to care for the new baby while your mother would return to work. By that point in my life I had abandoned any ambitions I once held about being a professional musician and had stumbled into journalism by writing feature articles about the arts for a smallish magazine. My thinking at that time was that this might lead on to bigger and better things. But I was working from home and so a switch in the traditional childcare arrangements made a great deal of sense. Even with the problems with the birth and your resulting condition, there never seemed to be sufficient reason to modify this original idea. So, I became, in the parlance of the early nineties, a househusband. Then a couple of years ago your mother and I separated and subsequently divorced. It has not been a particularly amicable parting but the fairly central issue of who you would live with was never really in any doubt.

I look at you and smile by way of a conclusion.

Shortly after, the nurse excuses herself but returns a few minutes later. She has a few more questions for us, some are about specific things like education, some are more general enquiries. Then, finally, she teeters, she falters and eventually succumbs. She asks me how I cope.

I am tempted to answer flippantly, tempted to reply that I depend entirely on a varying combination of caffeine, painkillers, self-righteousness and sarcasm. But in my experience hospitals tend to discourage flippancy. So I simply respond to her enquiry honestly.

Because you are my daughter, I tell her.

Because I love you.

And because sometimes I believe that it's probably the only thing I've ever done with my life that's been worthwhile.

This seems to satisfy her curiosity and we don't see her for the rest of the evening.

At bedtime we take our regular nightly trip on what we have

started to call the Wishboat. Once again, on your instructions, I steer it through the streets of Paris from the Gare du Nord down broad leafy boulevards, past all the places that we remember from our visits in the past. We cross the river over Pont Neuf and tonight we anchor our Wishboat at a café on the Left Bank where we sit together and watch the world go by.

Your eyes are closing but you are still awake and so I tell you that our little game, which I have come to rely on so much this past week, has started me thinking. I tell you that when I was about your age I used to ride my bike a lot. This was when I used to live in Cardiff and I used to cycle to school and cycle to see my friends. I inform you that for a great many years I was firmly of the opinion that I did my best thinking when I was cycling. I really did believe that my mind was clearer and I could think through problems and come up with ideas, plots and strategies far better when I was on my bike.

I had good reason to recall this when I was cycling back to the hospital earlier today through the all too familiar suburbs of South East London. Through neighbourhoods that have been my home for the past 16 years. For no particular reason I had started to think about the Wishboat. Then suddenly, without preamble or warning, a question half formed itself in my mind. It's a modified version of the same question that once manifested itself all those years ago as I pedalled my Halfords' Gemini 22 home through the outskirts of Cardiff.

Maybe it is not actually a tangible question; perhaps it's simply a vague unease, a momentary doubt or a wavering certainty. Maybe it's just another awakening of some sort. (A two-wheeled *satori*?) But for a minute or two, our everyday safe environment takes on a curious impermanence and that normally fixed sense of identity and of role and place succumb to a fleeting disquietude. The notion of home is suddenly flexible and the future feels less rigidly defined.

It is not a negative or unpleasant sensation in any way and although it passes swiftly, something of it lingers and nags at the back of the mind. Such moments occur quite rarely during a lifetime but around you they seem to happen fairly regularly.

But you have at this point drifted off to sleep and so I steal away to my mattress on the floor and leave you to your dreams.

The family (a collective nomenclature of convenience in this instance to refer to your grandma, your stepmother, your stepsister and your stepbrother) have now returned from Venice and over the next few days we are submerged in photographs, mementos and anecdotes. I am happy to see them and I quickly become familiar with the stabbing pangs of envy, which are my personal accompaniment to their stories.

There is something else too.

It is another sensation that defies easy definition yet it is one that I have experienced at fairly regular intervals these past 11 years and I am confident that it will pass in due course. It is another one of those things that I have usually assumed to be an inevitable side effect of the lives that you and I have had thrust upon us. It occurs half-way through the second batch of photos and I try once again to find the word. Not as powerful as isolation but it's hard to categorise, the Lido at dusk, a gondola. A nagging sense of detachment certainly, that vague feeling of being somehow perpetually *otherwise*, another shot of St Mark's Square, another gondola...

We make our way to the end of the final batch of photos and fairly soon, with some relief, I am once again explaining the underlying principles of traction.

You are eleven years and 119 days old and we are now in our fourth week in hospital. Your leg, we are told by the consultant who examines you today, is healing exactly as it should be. There have been no further problems or complications and everyone is pleased with your progress. He confirms that the pain is now obviously being well managed and I cast you a sly secret glance in preference to elaborating any further on the subject of Wishboats and our nightly voyages. I fear that the world of medicine is not quite ready for such things. But I chat to the consultant for a while and he confirms that the next stage will be re-plastering your leg into a sort of brace, after which we will be able to go home. This he anticipates happening in about a fortnight.

This is great news and for a few hours I feel elated at the prospect. For did I not once write in bold letters FREE THE SIDCUP TWO on the little whiteboard outside our little room? (Well, I'm told it amused the cleaning staff, it cheered me up too and it wasn't as if the board was being used for anything else.) But as our day moves towards its inevitable final moments I am surprised, stunned even, to discover that my joy has been tempered with a slight ambivalence.

Remarkably, there is a sadness.

Part of me is anxious to attribute this to possible over-tiredness, general fatigue and the resulting unwelcome side-effects. Well, we have rather been stuck in one room for almost a month. But that can only be a partial explanation. As the sky darkens over our private harbour and once more we prepare to embark on our travels, it slowly occurs to me how much this caravan-like existence has been of benefit to us. In the magnolia minimalism of this environment, somehow everything has been set in context once again. Hospitals inevitably have this effect but I make a promise to you and to me that when we leave we will take something of this time with us.

I suppose I might view this whole episode as a timely reminder of a life that both constrains and liberates, frustrates and inspires every second of every day. Nothing was ever spoken, nothing so melodramatically crass ever passed between us, but in some way I would like to regard certain elements of our lives as an inevitable consequence of a private, silent agreement.

Eleven years ago, against fairly overwhelming odds you survived, not unscathed, not unharmed but you survived. It is far easier to appraise with a decade's hindsight the extent to which you fought and fought just to hang on to life. The most fundamental yet sometimes the most powerful assertion of all human rights – the affirmation of the first person singular, 'I am'. That was your half of the bargain, mine was based largely upon the privilege of being a witness to those first months, the daily experience of awe, pride, gratitude and a whole muddled collection of feelings for which there are no words in any dictionary or in any language. My role, I now realise, has partly been to ensure that your fight was worth it, in short, that you made the right decision.

To this end I try to ensure that each day is fulfilling and worthwhile and by this means alone your life will ultimately be judged to be meaningful. I can see this now so clearly and I can see this as the true structure and framework to our lives. I don't feel that I have broken my promise to you and I'm not confessing to defeat or negligence in any way, only that maybe I need to sometimes be reminded of how sustaining, how reciprocal our little arrangement is.

The Wishboat heads eastwards and docks this evening in the Jardin des Tuileries where you drift to sleep beneath a tree in the warm evening sun.

From our portable CD player on the windowsill Muddy Waters sings pertinently (and not without a certain irony) 'I Feel Like Going Home'. Meanwhile, as I prepare myself for another night on the floor, the thoughts that have been circulating in my mind since that bike ride a week or so ago gather themselves once again. In the light of our stay here reaching its end, they herd themselves this evening into a series of questions. Questions that I now feel I must seek answers to.

According to the terms of our agreement.

You are six weeks old and finally I allow myself to accept the fact that you are coming home. I am elated and delighted obviously but fall victim at fairly regular intervals to the inevitable anxieties.

When I think of the responsibility.

When I think of what the future holds for you.

When I think of your condition.

When I think how it will change my life.

When I think of all that uncertainty.

A great panic passes over me and I just start to doubt my own strength and my own abilities. But all I have to do at those moments is look at you and I know that we're going to be all right. It only takes a few seconds and the fear passes. Everything is fine again.

If you gaze at *Uncertainty* long enough from a particular angle it eventually becomes *Not Predetermined* and turns itself into something infinitely more appealing. In this respect I can speak with a certain degree of authority as I've been gazing at it rather a lot recently.

You are not happy today and while I'm relieved that finally you seem able to cry nowadays, you do seem particularly miserable at the moment. You have started exhibiting jerky movements and while I'm assured this is not uncommon in children with what they are now terming your 'range of difficulties', I confess that it is unsettling to witness. However, the staff are still confident that you'll be leaving hospital in a few days.

Late in the day these jerking motions subside and you drift off to sleep for ten minutes. I take the opportunity to have a quick chat to the nurses. In doing so, I make no reference to the fact that I feel terribly self-conscious at the moment, almost shy, for want of a better word. As if I have been far too *exposed* around them. I feel as though I should be apologising to everyone.

The SCBU has been the venue for what is undoubtedly the single greatest trauma of my life. It has seen me in that raw, stripped, vulnerable (decidedly non-English) state. Now it is drawing to a conclusion and it feels very strange to be leaving it all behind – it is like the feeling that you've been talking too much and sharing too many confidences with a fleeting acquaintance.

Very odd.

Like sharing all your innermost thoughts and fears with someone you sit next to on the bus.

Over the next couple of days your mother and I get your room ready for you; it was decided that this should be delayed until it was absolutely certain that you would be leaving hospital. I return to the SCBU at least twice every day to see you and check on your progress. I tell you that your room is ready and waiting for you and that I hope you like it.

At one point I encounter the paediatrician and we sit together and discuss the various therapists and health visitors who are scheduled to call on us in the next few days. He tells me that you are a remarkable little girl and although I refrain from asking him directly to speculate on your future, he says simply that it would be in everyone's interest to keep an open mind. I thank him for all his help and return to your cot. As I'm leaving, I am surprised, in this domain of the universal 'Mum' and 'Dad', to hear him call me by my Christian name.

'Mark,' he says, 'so much now depends on stimulation. Sophie will need it now.' He pauses and then smiles at me. 'Good luck.'

You are six weeks and 3 days old and I take a photograph of your mother carrying you over the front step. It is a perfect moment and I resist all desire to reflect and speculate. Not now, not at this time. I want to enjoy this moment only for what it is.

A moment.

A season now passes and a season commences.

You are eleven years and 131 days old and your leg is currently being re-set and encased in plaster again. You endure this ordeal

with commendable fortitude. Meanwhile, I sit beside you and observe the process with interest. It has been difficult not to enjoy something so effortlessly primitive, so spectacularly low-tech as the whole treatment of fractures. I think it sort of reassures the secret Luddite in me.

The old fellow engaged in the actual plastering chats to me – his actual title is probably Fracture Technician or something of that nature and so I hesitate from referring to him as a plasterer. He asks me at one point what's wrong with you and I'm tempted to reply with all the incredulity I can muster that obviously you've broken your leg. But at the last minute cowardice or expediency gets the better of me and I tell him what I presume he wishes to hear. Your stepmother is infinitely better than I in these situations; she is far more fearless and quick-witted. On occasions in the past, in response to similar enquiries, she has answered without missing a beat that you have cerebral palsy but there's nothing *wrong* with you in the slightest!

That usually does the trick.

We return to our room where we wait to see a doctor. The afternoon passes slowly and when we eventually see him he examines your leg and the plaster brace, a structure that will ensure the bone heals correctly. He asks me a couple of questions and then says we can go home. Unfortunately it is now too late to arrange an ambulance and there is a strict protocol about children with fractures being discharged in this manner and so it will be ordered for the morning.

I gather our things together; I take down all your get-well cards, pack away all our books and sort out all your CDs. As the afternoon reluctantly surrenders itself to evening, the Wishboat embarks on its scheduled voyage. It travels terribly slowly this evening and you try and keep yourself awake as though you want the journey to continue. Tonight is therefore one of those rare occasions when I think that I know exactly how you feel.

In the morning a porter comes to collect us and I take one

final look at our room as I help manoeuvre your bed back out into the ward. I hold your hand as we travel down in the lift together. Happy to be going home. Of course we are happy to be going home. Although the past weeks have shown me that the notion of 'home' is a fairly flexible concept. Home is not an address, a postcode, a country, a neighbourhood or even a building. It is simply proximity to the person you love.

In the past month or so I have realised that home is something we will always be able to take with us.

I cannot make a specific promise to you this time because I do not want to disappoint you. Actually, I make it a habit never to disappoint anyone whose lower half is encased in plaster.

The ambulance pulls out of the hospital car park and joins the morning traffic on the bypass.

But I promise you that I will do my best.

And meanwhile I look through the rear window as I watch another season passing and a season commencing.

Second Season

The Same But Different

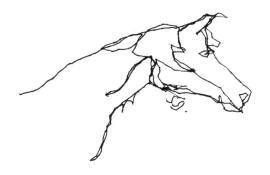

You are three months and 9 days old and the day about which I have dreamt for so long finally dawns. With little ceremony or anything to mark the moment, beyond a glance at the clock, at about quarter past eight this morning your mother sets off for her first day back at work. She says goodbye, kisses you and leaves us on our own.

I look at you for a few moments, gazing absently at breakfast TV and suddenly quite out of nowhere, if only for a couple of nanoseconds, I sense that I am beginning to panic.

It is a nebulous sensation, might be marooned, adrift or even abandoned.

But definitely *alone*.

Except that I am so conspicuously not alone any more.

Ever since you first left hospital I have so often thought about this moment. The past couple of months have not passed entirely without incident but all the while I have remained entirely focused on the day that your mother would return to work and we would start what Lou Reed calls our 'great adventure'. The day I would become a ... well, your health visitor calls us 'houseparents' but I confess I care little for the term and the physiotherapist referred the other day to 'main time carers'.

And so it begins.

It is a beautiful August morning and I decide that we should go out for a stroll for a couple of hours before it gets too hot. I chat to you about our plans for the day as I put you in your harness and we head towards the park. I remind you that this is a very important day for the both of us. It's a new era, I explain, just the two of us, you and me, father and daughter (apart from evenings and bits of the weekends, of course).

43

Today I notice all the other young mothers with their babies in prams and buggies. Every mother in the world seems to be out in the park today taking advantage of the early morning sun. I feel a certain affinity but it is no more than superficial.

Same but different.

So we find ourselves a nice big tree to sit under and I take you out of your harness. We sit listening to the birds. I rest my cheek against the top of your head and inhale your beautiful pure baby smell while I point out the birds to you and tell you the names of the ones I know.

I find a space in between my words and I leave us there for a second; you and I, our tree, the birds, the sun and the sky, as the significance of another moment passes over me. In recent weeks I realise that my mind has been operating along a very curious train of logic. One that would suggest that by remaining ignorant, by not knowing anything for certain one way or another, a person might find true *possibility*. And through recognising possibility I find that I am able to maintain a fairly positive outlook.

Same but different.

I have also discovered that everyone in the world it seems is an expert on child development. Everyone, that is, except me.

Sometimes I force myself to listen.

But usually I force myself not to.

It is perhaps to my advantage that since ceasing to actually be a child, you are the first child that I have spent any time with. Thus I have no means of making comparisons and judgements, you are you and I observe and scrutinise everything that you do uncertain of what is important or relevant.

There are obviously 'problems', you are often extremely stiff, you have very little movement at all and a particular way of staring at me sometimes, which still chills me to my very core. But you make a noise by clicking your tongue against the roof of your mouth and by this means sometimes we have a 'conversation' and I can soothe you back to sleep, or keep you comforted for a couple of seconds while I am out of sight. This suggests to me that something is definitely working in there.

What I am finding difficult is that most landmarks in child development are physical ones or the visible physical manifestations of mental ones. This makes it especially difficult for a mentally alert child with severe physical problems (I caught myself saying *children like Sophie* the other day – I must watch this, it's the sort of thinking I must try to avoid if at all possible). Making clicking noises, a most basic and primitive means of communication, has no official textbook status, it is not holding a cup or tracking a toy and thus means nothing to anybody except me.

However, I think it's brilliant and keep telling you!

Same but different.

And so my thoughts wander and I find myself thinking about faith again and often nowadays I remember the conversation I had with the nurse in SCBU, when she said that she considered faith more important than love. Perhaps she is right and perhaps it is that simple.

Meanwhile, you have started crying. It's time we were heading home again. I put you back in your harness and our return journey is undertaken at a noticeably increased pace.

Since I became A Person in My Situation, even the most well-meaning friends and family members are periodically prone to assumptions and generalisations. There is no malice in this and I imagine it must be very difficult for them sometimes. For example, I regularly find myself reassuring people that I *am coping*. This is generally my polite response to what I consider to be invariably an invalid or rhetorical question. To enquire if I am coping suggests that on some level I might be offered a choice in the matter – that at a point in the future I might possibly decide that I no longer wish to cope. It is a ludicrous proposition. Yes, I am coping, I tell them but whether or not they believe me is another matter.

The other subject that crops up regularly nowadays, in light, I imagine, of your mother and I deciding that we should take legal action against the Health Authority for the 'mismanagement' of your birth, concerns the level and intensity of my presumed anger. It seems that it is widely assumed that I must be incredibly angry about the events in the delivery suite that afternoon and the resulting situation. This is a much trickier issue and I don't really have an answer. Although I do understand how such a conclusion can be drawn, in fact I would make the precise same supposition about any person in my circumstances. So instead of offering a direct answer, I usually avoid the subject altogether by saying simply that I'm not nearly as angry about things as you are! That usually curtails the enquiries but I know that it's not actually addressing the question.

The decision to make a case out of your injuries is to ensure that you will have the resources for all the help you will need when you are older; I don't know if this can be actually regarded as vengeance or catharsis. In the SCBU all those months ago, there were often conversations with the staff about 'channelling anger' and I presumed then, as I do now, that these were the channels they had in mind.

But the truth is I don't actually think that I am angry; perhaps I should qualify that and add that it's not a particularly dominant emotion any more. A consequence of anger is that it tends to concentrate the mind, equally it has a tendency to mask and simplify issues. I'm sure that it's in there on some fundamental level but when I'm with you and it's just the two of us, I can't possibly imagine what use it could serve. I am aware that there is a doctor somewhere who 'mismanaged' your delivery, who is, by extension, possibly responsible for your condition, but directing anger, like directing blame, only serves to shift the focus and the emphasis away from you. I don't want to waste a single moment of the time we have thinking about him. That would be an even graver injustice. You are the most important person in my life now and I intend for that to remain the case. So I should endeavour to ensure that this doesn't get diverted by some mad vindictive urge for personal retribution.

With every molecule of your being, you fought so hard and struggled minute by minute, day by day, for the first six weeks of your life just for the chance to be here. As it stands now and as I imagine it will stand in future, I am guided by the principle that I was spared the unspeakable pain of your leaving. How can any man be this grateful, how could he love you as much as I do and even entertain notions about 'channelling anger'? How could I ever look at your beautiful little face or listen to you making your clicking noise and ever wish for things to be different? It's an utter irrelevancy as far as I'm concerned. We're a team now, you and I; we can't waste our time on such silliness. My anger would, in this context, be little more than an indulgence. It would be something that divided us and kept us apart. You would be less of a person with needs and hopes and more an 'issue', or a 'principle' about which I got angry. But you are so much more than that.

We've got things to do, we've got plans.

Same but different.

Over the following weeks, our days slowly form themselves into some sort of order and a routine is established. I realise that there is of course something deeply therapeutic about this and the implications are all but unavoidable. At a time of personal anxiety or crisis, the establishment of set patterns and structures to the day is of great benefit. It takes me a while to fully appreciate this but eventually I see that having a fairly rigorous daily schedule does afford me the chance to reclaim the tiniest suggestion of control in my life. It may seem a little obvious perhaps but at certain times one can be forgiven for the odd lapse.

I take you to the clinic for your regular check-up and while you are still very small and underweight for your age, you have actually gained a few ounces and so everyone is pleased. We

47

sit in the waiting-room and are gawped at quite unselfconsciously by a number of the other mothers there. I don't know if it's you or me that so piques their interest but it's a depressing interlude. One so often imagines that at such times one would feel a great surging sense of defiance, the bold stance of the unjustly exiled or the wrongly accused, that one would turn on them and confront their ignorance with a great speech that would reduce them all to tears of remorse. But sadly, it doesn't happen like that. I just find the whole thing deeply saddening and I whisper in your ear that the reason they are all staring at you is because you are the most beautiful girl they have ever seen in their dull, colourless lives.

I would imagine that the amount of care required by a three-month-old baby with problems is not appreciably any different to the amount required by one without problems. So, how about a little gesture of solidarity, ladies?

Same but different.

We make our way home with you crying and me muttering to myself.

You are four months and 2 days old and we return to the hospital for an out-patients appointment with your paediatrician. I must confess that I approach the meeting with certain trepidation but I am pleasantly surprised. First he confirms what I have suspected for a while now – that you are no longer having fits. Furthermore, he thinks that in some aspects of your development you are 'about where you should be'. He doesn't elaborate which aspects he has in mind but he is keen to stress the 'major physical problems' again so I sort of work it out for myself.

He confesses that he had been dubious about your chances of survival during those first few days and nights (and days and nights and days and nights) – the actual term he uses is 'not pulling through' – but he says he has been very impressed with your progress.

'Wait a minute,' he says as we're leaving, 'have you been given one of these?' With casual aplomb, he hands me a small book entitled *Your Child Has Cerebral Palsy*. Suddenly I feel as though the diagnosis has just been made official.

'So, that's the final verdict then?' I pout mirthlessly but your paediatrician just smiles and says nothing. He doesn't need to.

It is the instantly recognisable smile of someone recently unencumbered of bad news.

You have cerebral palsy.

You *have* cerebral palsy.

To cheer myself on the way home I tell you that we have just been part of an interesting new experiment. I explain that the BMA, in order to cut down on the stress that doctors experience, has just started this daring new initiative. Instead of having to pass on bad news to patients now, they simply hand over an informative booklet, which tackles the issue on their behalf. There is probably someone at our local health centre at this very moment being given a copy of, a copy of...

But it doesn't work and I arrive home in particularly low spirits.

You have cerebral palsy.

You *have* cerebral palsy.

I don't know what I was expecting, maybe I should have simply familiarised myself with the nomenclature by this point, maybe I was just hanging on to some vague thread of an idea I was too scared to even acknowledge or vocalise. Alternatively, perhaps I was simply trying not to think about it too much. This afternoon the terms were defined, the boundaries were set and restrictions and limitations permanently established. The future has just been modified, processed, realigned and is currently located within the pages of a small helpful leaflet. I know that we must accept this, I also know that it might be a bit of a struggle. However, I console myself in the knowledge that it is nothing compared to certain other struggles I have witnessed in the past few months.

Later in the evening after you've gone to bed I finally force myself to flick through the pages of *Your Child Has Cerebral Palsy*. When the little book sticks to the facts it is fine. I learn that, in simple terms, cerebral palsy is a condition that scrambles the messages between the brain and the muscles, causing stiffness (spasticity) and problems with movement and co-ordination. It can also cause problems with eyesight, hearing, speech and learning. Many cases result from problems during labour and birth and something like one in four hundred babies are affected.

The facts are fine.

There is no real reason to take issue with the pictures either, page after page of nice, clean, improbably happy smiling well-adjusted middle-class people enjoying quality time with their disabled child.

But later in the text when I read that 'fathers find it harder to cope' I must confess I do get rather irritated and in fact I tear the offending page out.

I would hate for you ever to see something like that.

The following morning I wake up with a headache, which barely qualifies as a surprise and you are in a particularly fractious mood for some reason. Breakfast is a struggle from start to finish and a long day stretches out in front of us. As your mother is leaving for work, I raise the question of a father's capacity to cope. She replies by simply enquiring about the source of this particular snippet of information and it is only after she has left that I realise that she didn't actually answer my question.

I try not to think about it all morning, then get annoyed with myself for trying to avoid the issues. Alternatively, I worry that I'm going to let the whole thing get on top of me and I'll just lapse into negativity and misery. We need some fresh air and inspiration, I tell you, and while you cry and complain all the way through, I get you dressed and put you in the harness.

It is a warm September day and we walk through the park with no particular destination in mind. You eventually cheer up and stop crying. Shortly afterwards, and possibly as a direct consequence of this, my headache lifts. By this point we have made our way as far as the market and I spend a distracted ten minutes or so wandering around the stalls. You are due for another drink soon and so I start to think about returning home. I'll just have a quick look at the paperback stall, see if there's anything interesting. I scan the titles on the spines but there's nothing of any immediate interest to me. But then I notice in amongst all the Barbara Cartlands and James Clavells, an old tatty pulp paperback edition of Pascal's *Pensées*. I tell you that this was a chap who knew a thing or two about faith, and on a whim I hand over two quid for the book.

I leave the book in my pocket and forget about it for the rest of the day. But late in the evening as I'm sitting with you in your room waiting for you to settle, I retrieve the book and idly scan a few pages at random. I come across a line that translates roughly as:

'It is impossible to have good reasons for not believing in miracles.'

For the first time all day I feel myself smiling.

You are eleven years and 146 days old and slowly we are adapting to life back at home again. You are still in plaster and we remain, as a consequence, more or less housebound, although we do manage a few hours in the garden each day. I am still sleeping downstairs next to your room where I can hear you in the night if you disturb and are uncomfortable. Sadly, the novelty of being in plaster has obviously started to wear a little thin and on a couple of occasions the Wishboat has been dragged out of its dry dock. The pain is under control now, the tedium, however, is proving more problematic. But by these infrequent nocturnal episodes I am able to keep alive certain aspects of that curious altered ambience we experienced when we were in hospital.

It's an odd and possibly even slightly alarming confession but I would have to concede that I do still miss elements of our time in Sidcup General. It brought to my attention that we continue to function better in our own little world, regardless of how depressing or unhealthy that may sound. We are able to set our own perimeters and limitations, work towards our own aspirations and goals and just generally get on with things in our own way and in our own time. Back in the real world with all its attendant distractions and considerations, promises can be so easily forgotten. In order to prevent this happening I make an appointment to see your solicitor as soon as possible.

This has started me thinking.

I would be the first to concede that there are so many disadvantages to a life spent at the margins but very occasionally things do turn in our favour. For example, a certain pleasure can be derived in the knowledge that our dreams and most heartfelt desires and enthusiasms are no longer restricted, no longer confined to what is considered safe or appropriate, no longer dictated to us by the whims of commerce or culture. We are free to ignore all the usual sensible choices, the careful decisions, the dreaded must-have items and replace them with our own notions and ideas. Ideas that might challenge, transcend or simply ignore the orthodoxy of these dreary constraints.

When nothing is certain, nothing is beyond us.

Same but different.

Meanwhile, I am trying to keep you occupied as best I can but your frustration is becoming more evident by the day. As you still cannot be transported anywhere, school is still obviously out of the question but your home tutor visits a couple of days a week and this puts a couple of nice neat holes in the general ennui. As always, you do enjoy these lessons but it's generally agreed that you tire quite easily at the moment. This is hardly a surprise but, as a result of this, it is decided to trim an hour or so off the afternoon sessions.

Also, the great delight you normally derive from selecting clothes from your ever–increasing wardrobe is no longer possible. Every day I have to make a selection from the same couple of skirts that are ample enough to accommodate the plaster.

You are going to sleep a little earlier than usual but I put this down to the mind-numbing boredom of the days.

The night before I am due to see your solicitor, I am sitting in my office at the front of the house, listening out to make sure you're suitably deep asleep and running through what I am going to say during the meeting. I have just finished scribbling a couple of lines in my diary. (I'm probably far too old to be keeping a diary but *journal* always sounds so hideously self-important.) I'd been thinking about this whole notion of escape and just jotting down ideas as they came to me. In any situation where one might find oneself dreaming of escape, what is the significant aspect? What one is escaping from? Whatever it might be that they are escaping to? Or is it the actual physical activity of the escape itself? Are they all indivisible elements of the same thing? Or does it vary from example to example?

Then, softly, I hear the distinct regular breathing pattern that means that you have finally fallen into a deep sleep and I decide that it's just one of those imponderable questions and that I should just go to bed.

Then it happens.

No warning.

No preamble.

From what little I remember of my RE lessons all those years ago, there's that story about God appearing to Moses as a burning bush and the tale of Saint Paul on the road to Damascus; when God is revealed to him by means of a great bolt of light. Fire and bright light in these cases being, I imagine, a way of representing a great spiritual awakening. I presume that this is possibly the route by which the word 'illumination' arrived at its twin meanings. A moment of clarity, a moment of revelation.

My personal experience this evening was less divine in origin but I must confess there was a particular stark drama to it, from which I derived a certain personal relevance. At just after eleven o'clock, the whole room is suddenly bathed in a faint orange glow as I see through the open curtains that, on the opposite side of the road, a Ford Escort has just burst into flames. Luckily, there are no houses on that side of the road just the park railings. The car was unoccupied and I wasn't quick enough to see the person or persons responsible but I hear the sirens and presume the police are nearby.

I watch the conflagration for a few minutes and can only see it as the perfect symbolic motif for this period in my life. My own moment of revelation: the burning Ford Escort.

By the time the fire brigade arrives and extinguishes the fire, the flames are already dying but what I have just witnessed, depending on my frame of mind, either hardens the resolve or acts as a sort of celestial confirmation.

Either way, I go to bed in good spirits.

We both sleep well and the following morning after your breakfast I leave you in the company of your grandma while I take the train into town on my own. I realise that it is the first time we have been out of each other's company since we returned from hospital. I take a deep breath and make my way to Holborn, rehearsing my lines and thinking about Max Miller and Sigmund Freud.

Many years ago, sufficient for me not to recall it in too much detail, I read Freud's *Jokes and their Relation to the Unconscious*. It is a fascinating, thought-provoking study, suggesting that humour is not trivial or petty but a method by which our unconscious self reveals itself to us. Widely regarded as one of his most readable works, it was written at a time when Freud's powers were at their greatest and it remains one of the key texts in the study of psychology. That being said, however, it should be pointed out that most of the jokes are rather pathetic.

Yet the idea that in jokes and comedy we find metaphors for

the human condition, perfect symbolic representations of emotions and ideas is an appealing one (it certainly appeals to Woody Allen). As I sit on the train and worry about the meeting this morning I keep remembering a joke that Max Miller told, one that seems to perfectly encapsulate my state of mind on these occasions. I don't recall the exact wording but the gist of it is as follows:

A farmer is ploughing a field one day when suddenly his plough breaks. Oh dear, he thinks, but then he remembers that Charlie Smith who owns a nearby farm has got a plough and he will be able to borrow his. So, he sets off for the farm. As he walks he starts thinking about Charlie Smith. He remembers that he's not a very nice man; in fact he's rather mean. He keeps walking and thinking to himself. Actually, he's one of the meanest men for miles around; he's not the sort of chap who would loan a person anything. He keeps walking and walking and eventually he reaches the farm house, He knocks on the door and when Charlie Smith opens it, he looks him right between the eyes and says, 'You know what you can do with your plough, don't you?'

There is no single line, slogan, term or expression that more accurately summarises my particular mindset this morning as I sit on the tube running through increasingly negative scenarios.

Despite my misgivings and much to my surprise the meeting goes rather well. I bring your solicitor up-to-date with your progress and then inform him that we want to move. Initially he says nothing in response to this; he just nods amiably and scribbles a line or two on his foolscap pad. But before he is able to voice anything in the way of a comment I just blurt out the second part and inform him that we want to move to Paris. He continues writing for a moment and then stops. His first question is nothing like the one I had been expecting.

'And this is what Sophie really wants, is it?'

Of course, this is the one thing of which I am completely certain and I tell him that it is absolutely what you want, more than anything in the world. Then I go on to explain that we've been making regular trips for about four years and that from the first time you saw the place you have wanted to live there. You have always been incredibly consistent in this. In fact, your actual way of putting it used to be that your heart needs Paris.

Your solicitor brings up the issues of health, education and your fortnightly contact with your mother but I notice with some relief that he hasn't actually laughed or ridiculed the suggestion by this point. I explain that it is our intention to sell the house in London and with the money raised, buy an apartment in Paris and also somewhere in Kent, not too far away from the Eurostar terminal in Ashford. This means we would be able to maintain a home in England and that our journey times would be quicker.

This is quite by far the hardest part of the whole meeting and I am able to tolerate the silence that follows for no more than a couple of seconds before I start to babble on about house prices. I think I say something to the effect that I had done a little research on the subject and that we could easily divide the capital raised from the sale of the house into two equal halves and then be able to afford two properties.

He thinks for a moment and then tells me that he doesn't foresee any objections to this and he advises me to find an agent, as property in Paris is famously hard to come by. He says that it's all subject to approval but, in principle, we can go ahead and put the house on the market. Perhaps I was wrong to imagine that a move to Paris would prove problematic but I take great comfort in the fact that it's far from uncommon for disabled children and their families to relocate abroad nowadays. In essence, he tells me, a move to Paris would be no more difficult than a move to anywhere in the UK.

I thank him profusely and make my way home as quickly as I can to tell you the news.

At bedtime, largely on my insistence, the Wishboat sets sail for Paris. An objective observer might notice that our journey is crammed with infinitely more descriptive detail than usual. You are asleep within minutes.

You are five months and 18 days old and we have another disturbed night. Generally speaking, you are much happier during the days now but you are still awake most of the night. On a fairly average night, you'll wake about one or two o'clock and then be up until four or five. Then, if I'm lucky, I might get a chance to grab a couple of hours sleep before your mother goes off to work and I have to take over again.

Each night, the routine is the same. Rather than risk waking the breadwinner, I take you quietly into the lounge and there I occupy the two of us as well as I can.

Some nights for no particular reason it just hits me.

I feel like we're the only two people awake in the whole world. There is nothing outside moving or living, nothing beyond these four walls.

There is no one apart from the two of us. We are alone and usually I can derive a great joy and comfort from this, I seek and find in our solitude a great sense of continuity. A certainty. But then there are the other nights like tonight.

I hold you in my arms tonight and you stare blankly up at me and I wonder if I were to die tonight would you mourn? Would you remember? Would you even notice? It's just the squint, I tell myself, that's all, that's what makes your eyes go funny sometimes, you are tired too, you must be, you've been awake for hours...

What if I am wrong about everything?

How can I even think that?

How then could I look you in the eye?

These are the thoughts I share with no one.

I don't have to share them with you because you understand me.

One day, if I live to be an old man and I'm frail and have trouble walking, when I can't always control my bladder and I'm frightened. When I can no longer make myself understood and I'm being patronised with cocoa and trips to the seaside. When all my dignity has been eroded away to nothing, when I am degraded and inhuman, I just pray that my memory remains intact. Because it will recall a child's face and it will be your face as it is tonight. You will smile and wink at me.

We will be equals at last.

You've already been through all of this.

The following morning just as we're leaving for another outpatients' appointment, I receive a phone call from my editor. The piece I wrote about the painter Henry Fuseli is going in next month's magazine more or less as I wrote it. This is something that, I must confess, cheers me up enormously. So when he asks me if he can have 1,500 words on the Cabaret Voltaire by the end of the month I respond in the affirmative. I immediately regret this. With your sleep patterns at the moment, I realise that I should be far more hesitant about making commitments like this.

We have an earlier appointment this week and as a consequence manage to avoid the dismal spectacle of the staring gawping mothers. The meeting itself is fairly positive and your paediatrician seems once again reasonably happy with your progress. We talk for about ten minutes and it is gratifying to hear the odd note of cautious optimism drift into his conversation.

'She is very beautiful,' he says at one point and this sounds utterly genuine. So I tell him about your way of communicating with me and he smiles.

'Before communication,' he says, 'comes contact.'

He lets this hang in the air for a couple of seconds and I'm inclined to just let it dangle there on its own. The tone is reassuring, the words vague yet obviously well chosen and I wonder if he has used the phrase before.

We talk about your fits or rather the total absence of fits

58

nowadays and he agrees to me reducing and then stopping the last of your anti-convulsants. This is something I consider to be extremely good news and I feel we have taken another cautious step away from the days of the SCBU. As we are leaving I mention that you have not been in the best of moods this past week. He takes a quick look inside your mouth and confirms that you are teething.

Your first tooth.

In such a short, troubled life it is rather heartening to witness something so incredibly *ordinary*.

Although I suspect in future I will encounter innumerable incidents of this nature, in a way it is unsettling to be dragged back to the world from which I so often feel exiled.

Same but different.

You are six months and 26 days old and awake in the early hours of a day that will remain historic as the day Margaret Thatcher resigns. Later in the morning your mother and I set off for town and our first meeting with a solicitor. At least, I think to myself as I kiss you goodbye and leave you with your sitter, you have lived long enough to witness an important historical event and, by the way, ding-dong the wicked witch is dead!

This sadly proves to be the last cheerful moment in an otherwise largely dispiriting day. To be fair, I have been dreading this day ever since the moment that your mother and I first committed ourselves to making a claim against the health authority.

The day transpired to be every bit as difficult as I imagined.

This initial meeting is basically a chance for the solicitor to introduce himself and to take us through some of the procedures for which we are told we must be fully prepared. Some of it I find a little distressing. For one thing, I must confess that I had absolutely no idea that cases of this nature can often drag on for ten years.

Ten years!

We are, however, reassured that your case 'will probably be settled in half that time'. In simple terms, we are informed, your condition resulted solely from medical negligence and so those responsible for the negligence should be made accountable. Yours is, we are told, a relatively straightforward case and the firm has dealt with far more borderline cases in the past.

By about this point in the meeting I realise that I will need to keep these two versions of you absolutely separate. There is the you that I know and I love, the version that is familiar to me, the one that makes clicking noises and has a new tooth, the version that I will see at home later on after all this is over. The other version has exactly the same name and the same date of birth but I need to keep her distant and entirely apart from you. This alternative version I can more easily discuss with a solicitor, I can talk about the problems with development, growth, health, learning and all the uncertainties about the future but she's not you. Her eyes don't smile like yours, she doesn't like coming out with me in her harness and listening to me ranting on about everything and nothing in particular, and the top of her head doesn't have that milky smell that I love so much.

The solicitor concludes the meeting by stating in the most direct manner that it is imperative that your mother and I both remember that the claim is on *your* behalf. He clarifies the remark by saying that in order to get as far as a settlement or a trial we will have to relive the worst couple of hours of our lives over and over again to countless experts. If we don't focus our minds on the fact that we are going through it all for you, we will never last the distance, whatever the incentive. I will have people coming into our home over the next few years and all they will want to talk about will be those first hours.

Then you will be taken to appointments all over the country, to see 'experts' where I will have to sit and listen to all manner of damning judgements on you. Finally, I will also have to listen to people arguing about your life expectancy, which is very important because a large proportion of the claim is for your 'future lack of earnings'.

The shorter the expected life, the smaller the settlement!

I replay this simple equation in my mind over and over, astonished at its brutal barbarism and I leave the building in fairly low spirits.

Your mother goes off to work and I make a quick detour up Oxford Street to get you some warmer pyjamas and I am back home again by mid-afternoon.

The following day we are visited at home by your physiotherapist. She has been coming at fairly irregular intervals over the past couple of weeks but is now going to be calling at the same time each week. By means of a series of fleeting moments like this, I realise, I will begin to understand gradually, and slowly learn to work around your condition. I talk to her about the appointment with the solicitor, only because I imagine, on some psychological level, I need to talk to someone about it.

Then, as though seeking a positive alternative to this, I mention the little things, the subtle changes in your behaviour I have observed recently. Things that suggest to me that you are showing some cognitive development. I mention your clicking noises and that time you were rubbing your ear before we took you to the GP and he confirmed you had an ear infection. I mention the fact you seem to respond to specific types of music and that you will always look out for me whenever I enter a room. I babble on in this fashion for a few minutes until I realise she isn't saying anything. She simply smiles and nods. When she does speak she completely ignores all my previous remarks and asks me if I've been doing the exercises with you she had suggested during her previous visit.

This is my first inkling of what will become a major factor in the months and years to come. My first brush with the natural reticence of special needs professionals and my first lapse into, what is usually believed to be, fairly archetypal behaviour for parents in my situation.

There is, I imagine, a certain underlying truth to this particular stereotype, indeed it is mentioned in *Your Child Has Cerebral Palsy*. Parents are often unable to face up to the extent of their child's disabilities and as a consequence are often prone to deny them. Or more frequently, they will concentrate on isolated observations to which they might attach enormous positive significance. It's an understandable reluctance to face up to a particularly difficult situation and I realise, to the uninitiated, I am displaying certain orthodox tendencies in this regard.

However, this afternoon outlines a formula for countless conversations in the future. My observations are often deemed invalid simply because of a particularly rigorous equation that states that *some* parents can *sometimes* be in *denial*. But it is the supreme caveat and devastatingly effective! I feel I should say something in my defence but I just answer in the affirmative; yes, I have been doing the exercises with you.

Then she returns to the point I made earlier and asks what sort of music you like. I say that at the moment you like anything by Django Reinhardt but you only like doing your exercises to 'Lust For Life' by Iggy Pop.

She then asks me if I think you might like to try music therapy.

I wince at the word 'therapy' and silently rebuke myself. I say it might be interesting and she promises to make some enquiries.

You are eight months and 28 days old, it is Christmas Eve and I'm having a bad night.

It caught you at a bad angle, I keep telling myself, and on reflection I am probably speaking the truth.

But tonight, maybe for the first time since April, I come

62

close to that point of pure despair, at the very moment of surrendering myself for ever. I knew Christmas was going to be difficult, it is another one of those ordinary things that happen around you that only remind me how extraordinary our lives are.

According to your mother's German traditions we put the Christmas tree up this evening. When it is finished and looking suitably splendid, your grandad takes a couple of Polaroid photographs of you and your mother looking at all the decorations. An everyday, happy domestic scene but with a slight twist, your eyes stare upward with the pupils just about visible, while your mouth hangs open.

It is a face that tells you everything because it tells you nothing.

The Polaroids are left on the table when everyone goes to bed. I am the last one to leave and as I make my way out of the lounge I pick them up and glance at them. I look at your vacant expression and suddenly I am overpowered by a moment of absolute fear and despair. Like I will drown inwardly from all the tears I have blinked back. All the times I have wanted to scream and the times I have just wanted to wake up from this. I feel my heart pounding and it is as though at that moment I am experiencing the full extent of all the suppressed emotions of these past eight months concentrated into a couple of seconds. Just as I am beginning to wonder if I am about to die, or faint or pass out, the sensation passes.

I don't want to ever go through that again.

But like I say, it was probably just an unfortunate angle.

However, I am still feeling slightly subdued the following morning as we pass another small milestone in your life. Your first Christmas Day. We sit around the dining table opening our presents in the traditional manner. You are sitting on your grandma's lap. You are having one of your better mornings, I'm pleased to say, and being terribly well behaved.

Then, just as the final present has been opened and I am

preparing myself to start tidying up, in full view of everyone, you take a deep breath and SPEAK!

Obviously you do not speak in the traditional sense, but you produce this vast sentence of nonsense syllables, typical baby talk, which is, however, an accurate and perfect approximation of spoken English.

We were all dumbfounded, equally in awe, I presume, of your flair for dramatic timing as much as your vocal talents. But naturally, after last night, the joy I feel at this is multiplied a hundredfold. Your Christmas message this year is also a very private message from daughter to father.

For a moment or two you stare across the table at me and I feel suitably chastised.

'Thanks,' I whisper, 'sorry and er ... happy Christmas.'

You are eleven years and 193 days old and finally, after more months than I care to remember, you return to school. The plaster was removed from your leg about three weeks ago and we've been taking it all a little gently, just gradually easing you back into things. We've had a few home visits from your physiotherapist and an outpatients appointment at the hospital, and everyone seems happy with your rate of recovery. Today is a day I have thought about for such a long time, a day that seemed mystical and distant back in August. I suppose a return to school always marks a sort of official conclusion to the summer and in many ways today seems no different.

I accompany you into school in the morning and go for a chat with your head teacher. I had intended for this to simply be a means of bringing the school up-to-date with what's been happening to you. But it transpires that our meeting takes on a significance that I had not hitherto anticipated. Before its conclusion, it also occurs to me that this is probably the last time that I will see the inside of his office.

We chat about your accident for a while, he tells me about

his latest plans for the school and then I manage to steer the conversation towards the purpose of my visit. I tell him that you and I are going to be moving in the near future.

I am certain that I detect a fleeting expression of relief on his face and I wouldn't blame him. In fairness to him he manages to ask 'when?' rather than 'how soon?' and I explain the situation to him. Despite his becoming, in recent years, a fairly impressive personification of my perceptions of authority and opposition, I do have a certain respect for the man. Sometimes I like to fool myself that this might be mutual. But this is not to suggest I am unaware that we have been at loggerheads at times in the past.

We talk amiably about your accomplishments at the school and all the great things that you've done over the past few years. There seems to be a degree of genuine pride in your achievements and the controversy that once raged about your intelligence and your abilities now seems part of the unconnected distant past. It was a controversy that was resolved in your favour finally by a few brave souls within a stone's throw of this very office.

At one point, he reminds me of our first meeting, when I had said, rather grandly on reflection, that if I was wrong about you then we really will have lost very little, but just imagine what we will have achieved if I am proved right. I smile at the recollection but I would still stand by those sentiments. Although perhaps phrased a little less obviously.

I tell him that we will hopefully be relocating 'somewhere in Kent' and we chat about future education plans for you. As virtually all your academic input is now overseen by your personal tutors, I say that I am confident that at least that side of things will continue without any major changes. I remind him that you have the provision of a permanent tutor for one day a week written into your Statement of Special Educational Needs. This has put you in a virtually unique position. I'm pretty certain he doesn't need reminding of this but I just thought I'd slip it in to the conversation. I also mention that we are also trying to get a place in Paris but this is all but ignored in favour of a brief résumé of the building work he is intending to have done at the school.

Then, as I'm preparing myself to leave, he introduces into the conversation a word that has never been uttered previously in my company. It gives the whole meeting a magnitude that transcends our previously trivial discussion about traction and relocation.

He tells me that I will have to start thinking about some *accreditation* for you before too long. It would be better to make some long-term plans at this stage. I nod automatically at this but the reality is that I have never given a moment's thought to accreditation or any sort of qualifications for you for that matter.

Having thrown a gauntlet across the desk in my direction, he feels no great compunction to shake my hand as I leave his office.

I return home thinking about this, mulling it over in my mind over and over again. Of course he is absolutely right, I should start to at least think about the next few years and what possibilities are out there for you. Slowly, I calm down and reflect upon the conversation and consider why I found it so unsettling, for I did find it unsettling. I can only assume that it's the realisation that all we've been through thus far is only a part of a much longer process.

That what we have achieved in the past couple of years is transitional rather than definitive.

The old equation, as I believed it to be until earlier this morning, constituted just two points on a single line:

FAITH – CONFIRMATION

Now I realise how naïve I have been. There are not two points but three and the equation is subtle and infinitely more complex. It goes something like this:

66

UNCONDITIONAL FAITH – CONDITIONAL FAITH – PROOF

Alas, I realise I have been fooling myself into thinking we had reached any sort of conclusion; we have only reached the second stage. As far as faith is concerned, its resolution in academic terms is not confirmation but proof. The sooner I accept this and work towards it, the better. I don't know whether I should thank him for this or not. I suppose it needed to be said and I needed to hear it but I have a few dark, desperate SCBU hours in the afternoon until you return from school.

After more than a decade in your company and all the familiarity that would imply, I fool myself that I've become reasonably adept at reading your different moods. Daily contact with someone who has no speech whatsoever does tend to encourage the development of such a skill. Over the years, I have learned that a person's face actually requires very little mobility to be infinitely expressive and I can usually distinguish a dozen or so subtly different variations in your countenance. But then there are days like today when you seem distant and as enigmatic as any human being can. I ask you about this after I've given you your drink. Tiredness, I conclude, is the probable cause but I do wonder if I'm witnessing something else today. I've been in similar situations myself over the years and it might be that great sudden moment of awareness: that you are no longer where you would wish yourself to be. I suppose it is simply the natural impatience of the young; sometimes it's too easy to forget what that is like.

If this is the case then there are still certain forces somewhere working for you because the following morning there arrives in the mail a letter from the Paris property agency I made enquiries with a while ago. It's a sort of detailed questionnaire about our precise requirements and our price range. I read through it with you as I'm feeding you your breakfast. You seem to be much happier this morning and I wonder if this is a good night's sleep, coincidence or the contents of the letter.

After your tutor arrives for your morning session I shut myself away to complete the questionnaire. It is far less complicated than I would have imagined. It is actually rather like writing a letter to Father Christmas. I state that ideally we would like a two-bedroom apartment, a fine old Haussmann period one would be nice. We would like a lift and, because of access to Eurostar, we would like it as close to the Gare du Nord as possible. Our budget is simply half the asking price for our current house, which goes on the market next week. And by the way, I've been a good boy all year and I always do as I'm told...

I walk around the corner and post the letter whereupon my ebullience suddenly collapses on me.

I start to think about your accreditation again and what a challenge that is going to be for you. Of course it would be the ultimate proof and the greatest vindication of all but do I really want to put that sort of pressure on you? I'm aware that it's no different to the pressure that will be on other teenagers in a few years time; it's just that you have so many other things to deal with on a daily basis.

There is, I quickly discover, a darker, more confessional aspect to this whole issue. The question of whether such an achievement is truly for *your* benefit, or might it possibly be for mine? Wouldn't this be the ultimate personal denouement? Is this the means by which we can stand up to all the people who ever doubted you? Or do I mean who ever doubted me? Words like vengeance, victory, vanquish and defeat, the lexicon of every battle-weary general, hover at the perimeters of this protracted dilemma and worry me all the way home.

They never said it was going to be easy. But it's never difficult in the ways you imagine it will be.

You are eleven years and 242 days old and we pass an oddly

subdued and largely uneventful Christmas Day. It is our first Christmas without my father/your grandad and it is every bit as tricky as I feared it might be.

Same but different.

All day I mull over a single thought in my mind. That this year of all years – the year of the dual airplane attacks on the World Trade Centre, my father's absence strikes a particularly poignant parallel. Like the Twin Towers (surely now the most famous thing in the world that isn't there), he seems to have taken on far greater significance and magnitude by no longer existing – a colossal space remains, infinitely larger than the one occupied during the lifetime.

This sensation of absence remains with me all day although it reaches a sort of peak over the lunch when I find myself unable to converse or even concentrate.

All day I have been wondering how you are coping and I realise that it must be difficult for you too. Your grandad's passing earlier in the year was your first encounter with the death of someone close to you and, although difficult to pin down precisely, I think it has had a subtle yet quite profound effect on you. It has most frequently manifested itself in trying to ensure that your grandma is all right and insisting that we go to see her every day. Also, that we take her with us whenever we go anywhere. Even now, this continues.

A day or so ago, you reminded me that we must be brave for Grandma, and once again I find that I am taking your words to heart.

At one point, shortly after lunch, in an attempt to alleviate the general mood, I take you out into the garden and we say happy Christmas to the oak tree that you and I planted as our own memorial to him back in the summer. It looks bare today, barren even. We look at the small plaque on which your simple choice of dedication reads:

BEST GRANDAD
2001

It gets cold and we return inside. As the afternoon progresses, we do all our usual Christmas things but truly there is very little pleasure to be had today. It is more a question of getting through the day and praying that next year's festivities are slightly easier.

Boxing Day continues along very similar lines and I'm grateful when we get to the evening and the end of the day is in sight. I'm in the process of getting your final drink of the day ready when the phone rings.

Of all the people you least expect to call you on Boxing Day, our Paris property agent must be fairly near the top of the list. He's calling from Paris and he sounds seasonally jolly. We exchange a few pleasantries and then it's down to business. He's found us an apartment! Simple as that. I am stunned by this news and can barely construct an appropriate response. Apart from a handwritten acknowledgement of the return of the questionnaire a couple of months ago, there has been no further contact until this phone call. Picking his way through my wordless exclamations of surprise and wonder, he tells me that he has found a property that perfectly matches our requirements and how soon can we get over to Paris to view it. He explains that we are not likely to find a similar apartment if we look for another year and property in Paris changes hands very quickly. I take a deep breath and I tell him I'll call him back.

I give you your drink and tell you what I've just been told. I realise you are tired and that it's been a fairly trying couple of days but I ask if you would like me to arrange a trip to Paris for us as soon as possible so that we can have a look at an apartment. Your expression is all the confirmation I need. I call the agent back and tell him that we will be over in a day or so and he implores me not to leave it any longer than that.

This evident urgency converts itself into a note of caution and I allow this to serve as a dampener on the enthusiasm of the moment. But I tidy up and wash up, imagining apartments in Paris and reflecting upon my father, Wishboats and next Christmas.

It's about midnight when I finally go to bed. On my way, I call in to see you, to check on you and to say goodnight. I shouldn't really register the slightest surprise at what I discover.

You are still wide awake and smiling to yourself.

You are eight months and 6 days old and, having survived Christmas, I feel equally triumphant at making it into a new year.

It wasn't that last year was that terrible, more that I simply wasn't prepared for it.

I spend this New Year's day in a sort of reflective stupor. I suppose it is unavoidable really. I think of myself and my life a year ago and picture such a charmed, easy existence. I was worrying about bills, if I should replace my computer, if my boots would last another winter, if I should read anything into the fact I didn't receive a Christmas card from whoever...

A massive silliness really.

Looking back, I see so much innocence and so little fear. But I also see a trivial life, an unfulfilled life, a life lacking substance or purpose, a life, in other words, without you.

Over the next few weeks or so you seem to be in a fairly permanent bad mood and there are times when I can feel myself nearing the point of losing my temper with you. I have shouted at you a couple of times when you seem to be carrying on unnecessarily. I remind you that I understand your anger and frustration but I am on your side and you shouldn't take it out on me.

Sometimes, I have to say, you respond very well to the occasional harsh word and you calm down very quickly. I take this to be a good thing but wouldn't wish to broadcast it particularly. I think being frustrated, which you are so evidently at times, is also a positive sign; it would suggest very strongly that you have an awareness on some level of your situation.

This particular period of our lives coincides with a lengthy piece about Rousseau I am supposed to be writing for the magazine, ostensibly to tie in with the publication of a new biography. It's dragging on and on and I keep shielding myself from phone calls enquiring of me when it will be finished. As this is entirely dependent upon your moods at the moment it is not a question I can answer. It's a difficult situation and not one I foresee being resolved in the near future.

One morning a welcome respite is provided by the postman. He delivers a letter from the Health Authority inviting us to attend an appointment at the Bardon Clinic in North London. I recall that your paediatrician had mentioned something about this place a while ago. It is a specialist centre for children with cerebral palsy and other similar disorders. The clinic has an exemplary record and reputation and apparently its results, I was told, are nothing far short of remarkable.

The letter explains that this initial appointment will be a consultation in the form of an assessment between the clinic, your physiotherapist, your paediatrician and the two of us. As the day of this consultation grows nearer, I hear over and over again of the high regard in which the clinic is held. Your physiotherapist, who drives us to the appointment, informs us on a number of occasions, 'their input could be very significant.'

As it turned out she was absolutely right, it was *very* significant but not in the way that either of us might have anticipated.

Firstly, we are kept waiting for three quarters of an hour and when the clinic's chief specialist finally makes her entrance I confess I take an instant dislike to her.

'Sorry I'm so late,' she says as she sweeps into the room.

Then she shouts a greeting at us, and the appointment spirals downwards from there.

It is an afternoon I know I will never forget. Today I remember it for all the wrong reasons. I pray that one day in the future you and I will remember it for all the right ones.

Firstly, the specialist tells me, after examining you for the briefest time, that the centre can do nothing for children with your 'complex problems'. Then she asks me if you recognise me when I walk into a room. I say that you seem to.

'But,' she barks, 'does she smile at you?'

'Er... no. Not always.'

'No, I don't expect she does. To be honest I doubt if she actually does recognise you.'

I find myself wondering, in amongst all the accolades that have been hurled in the Bardon Clinic's direction over the years, if there have been a great many for tact and sensitivity.

She then goes on to confidently inform me that you do not 'process information'. You have no way of understanding what you see or what you hear. Your brain is 'shut down' as she so charmingly puts it and you have negligible cognitive powers. This, she tells me, is unlikely to improve.

At this point, to his eternal credit, your paediatrician, who has been listening attentively to this exchange, speaks up on your behalf.

'Actually, I think Sophie has made a lot of progress in the last few months,' he says.

But no one is listening to him.

The specialist then places you in a high-backed chair and watches as you rub the back of your head against the head rest. She points out that this is your way of 'understanding your environment', of 'locating yourself'. By rubbing your head against the seat you are 'using a most primitive method of identifying your surroundings'.

I make eye contact with the paediatrician and experience a fleeting moment of camaraderie.

'Can I ask a question?' I ask the specialist.

'Please do.'

'You say Sophie can not process information.'

'That's right.'

'Nothing goes in.'

'Nothing whatsoever. Sorry.'

'So by what mental process exactly is she 'understanding her environment' as you put it? Even if it is by rubbing her head, how is that information turned into an understanding of her environment? By whichever way you look at it, there is some cognitive process at work, surely?'

The paediatrician gives me the briefest smile, which I flatter myself is an expression of support. Meanwhile the specialist points out in the time-honoured fashion that it would take far too long to explain.

'I suppose,' she says, 'in layman's terms it might appear that way but sadly it is not the case.'

The appointment reaches its grim finale with the specialist pulling and pushing you about in a manner that looks quite un-medical at times and reiterating that the clinic is unable to do anything for children like you. (Even in the marginalised, segregated world of the disabled, I am learning that there are still those who find themselves pushed to the edges even further.)

I leave the clinic in a state of simultaneous anger and deep depression. I realise now what needs to be done, I realise what responsibility rests upon my shoulders.

Belief and faith in you are fine in themselves but the real world requires evidence! And the burden of providing that evidence is probably down to me. I need to find a way of proving that you are mentally alert, which I *know* you are. But these people aren't interested in intuition, they want X-rays and graphs.

They want their evidence.

They know all about fathers not being able to face up to their children's disabilities. They wrote the book! And that is all I am in their eyes. Just another poor sad, deluded fool!

My confidence in you is, in their eyes, simply my denial of the problem.

A nice, simple equation but one that I must be on my guard against always.

We return home and I underplay the general trauma when your mother asks me about our afternoon. Interestingly, I later find some solace from the most unlikely of sources. On page 11 of *Your Child Has Cerebral Palsy*, I find a reference to the fact that most children with cerebral palsy have 'normal intelligence'.

Over the next couple of days, I confess I have a few bleak moments, when I feel that something has just been taken away from me.

Something very precious.

But I will get it back.

I promise you.

You are a year old today and the day threatens to crumble under the weight of its own significance. The day falls on a Saturday and people call in throughout the day with cards and presents. It's not a formal gathering in any sense of the word but I feel that the day has been marked. It is not easy buying something for a one-year-old under any circumstances and choosing something for someone with a very limited range of movements and abilities poses even more problems. Still, you have lots of new clothes and books and more cuddly toys than any self-respecting one-year-old could wish for. Somebody gives you your own CD of Lust For Life, which raises a few eyebrows from those not in the know.

A friend we haven't seen for a couple of weeks visits with her twin boys, three months old and both, I'm less than thrilled to learn, weighing more than you do at twelve months. We catch up on some news and she enquires about your progress.

Are you crawling at all?

Standing?

Are you sitting unsupported?

Are you babbling?

Each time I reply in the negative. I actually feel acutely sorry for our friend; the whole conversation was probably far more awkward for her than it was for me. Sadly, I am getting all too used to it.

The answer I want to give to all her questions is, of course, 'not yet' (I still enjoy that precious state of not knowing), but these are the thoughts I keep private.

Not for fear of sounding like a deluded parent.

But because I have no intention of putting any more pressure on you.

At intervals throughout the day I offer edited highlights of our trip to the Bardon Clinic; and the resulting emotions that its recall stirs in me have grown no easier in the past month or so.

As the afternoon is drawing to a close, I am alone in the kitchen making coffee for the masses when I glance at the clock.

It is half past five.

Then, suddenly without the slightest warning, I am reeling. One of those rare moments when one is simply overwhelmed by the blatantly obvious! Finally, just in the nick of time, it's hit me. It is a year ago to the minute, I think, to the very minute I first caught sight of something grey and lifeless and begged a nurse to tell me what was happening.

That was *exactly* a year ago.

How could I forget the significance of such a thing?

You have life.

You *still* have life.

You have fought so hard for every single solitary second of this year.

How dare I lose sight of this?

Every minute is a victory and every hour of every day is still a cause for celebration.

I return to the lounge where people are once again singing

'Happy Birthday' to you and I sense that now, with the passing of your first year, there is once again a gentle shift in the seasons.

You are eleven years and 251 days old and it is a cold morning in early January as we travel to Paris on Eurostar to view this apartment. You are a little sleepy during the journey but remain in predictably and excusably high spirits. I start to remind you that you shouldn't get over-excited and that we haven't even seen the place. I waste ten minutes or so in this fashion, generally advising caution, before it dawns on me I might be encouraging you to develop a sort of reasoning similar to mine: namely the Max Miller and The Plough mindset. I very quickly conclude that this would be an incredibly bad idea and so I instantly refrain. I leave you to the thrill of our adventure while I gaze absently out of the train window.

When we arrive at the Gare du Nord, we are met at the barrier by our agent. He is standing in the line of drivers and chauffeurs holding up a card that reads, 'WELCOME TO PARIS, SOPHIE'.

It's a well thought-out gesture, particularly as we haven't actually met face to face and it is one that I really appreciate. I have always taken very kindly to people who talk directly to you rather than largely ignoring you and asking me questions about you. It's a small courtesy and it saddens me greatly that it happens so rarely. I would readily concede that it is difficult talking to someone who can't talk back but it's not impossible and I always appreciate those who make the effort. Or those people who make an assumption of awareness or intelligence. Sadly, they are still very much in the minority.

We exchange the briefest pleasantries and then he instructs us to follow him. He walks quickly and, pushing you in your wheelchair, we struggle to keep up with him. Luckily, we are only following him for about a minute when he stops abruptly and points to the building on the opposite side of the street. 'There,' he says, proudly.

Despite our proximity to such a major rail terminal, we are standing in a remarkably quiet well-maintained little street and our attention is currently being marshalled towards a late nineteenth century four- or five-storey apartment block in the very typical Haussmann style of the period. From simply observing the exterior, even on such a dismal January morning, my heart begins to race.

After about ten minutes, we are met by the vendor and his agent and they take us into the building and, with the least possible ceremony, they show us around the apartment. As we look around I keep looking at your expression and recognise in the joy and wonder a fairly accurate approximation of my own feelings. I am simply older and slightly more adept at masking such things. There's a Latin quote from the *Satires of Horace* that I remember from school, *Hoc erat in votis*.

This is what I once longed for.

I can think of no better way of summarising our first few minutes in the apartment.

I am told the vendor wants a quick sale and, seeing that every room is literally crammed to bursting point with stuff, it is fairly easy to understand why. I take you into one of the rooms and tell you that this could be your bedroom. It has a wooden parquet floor, a beautiful marble fireplace with a mirror just about visible behind bunk beds, and it is wonderful beyond words.

Our agent puts his head around the door and reminds us that places like this at this price rarely come on to the market. He adds that although this is the first property that we've viewed, we are unlikely to find anything that better suits our needs if we were to see a dozen or a hundred apartments. He urges me to make a quick decision.

Naturally, my mind was made up on the street outside but obviously this is your decision too and I want your confirmation.

I pull out your notebook and put a pen in your hand. I ask you the simple question: do you want us to buy this apartment?

You are smiling and looking happier than I have seen you in months. It is therefore a surprise when, in your unmistakable spidery hand, you simply write:

no

You leave the pen on the paper as I register a level of shock and confusion. You heard what the agent just said and I am amazed that you would not want to live here, it is absolutely perfect. Isn't this exactly what the Wishboat was all about? I thought that it was all leading up to this minute, all our dreams and our plans, have I misread...

Then I watch as you simply add a letter:

now

Of course, it is just about possible that your arm is stiff today, or you are finding it difficult writing in different conditions from what you are used to. But I don't believe that. I see the smile on your face and I recognise a certain sense of mischief. You are completely aware of the situation and are simply enjoying the moment; just amusing yourself for a couple of seconds at our expense. I tell our agent that we want the apartment.

An hour or so later we are all sitting in the office of the vendor's agent on the Boulevard de Magenta and I am signing documents; the relative exoticism of the location successfully counterbalancing the abject tedium of the actual task. There is a seemingly endless pile of papers that require my signature. But after a couple of hours, the deed is done and I'm told that the apartment is ours and we can take possession in two months' time. I throw a puzzled expression roughly in the direction of our agent and he explains that this is how the process of conveyancing works in France. This is now a firm and binding contract between buyer and seller and it seems an infinitely simpler and less agonising process than the British equivalent.

Our business concluded for the day, we walk back to the Gare du Nord as the sun breaks through the clouds. Instantly, I interpret this as some sort of celestial confirmation that you and I have done the right thing.

I lean over and whisper something in your ear.

I tell you that the Wishboat has landed.

You are twelve years old and you wake up in Paris having just spent your first night in our new apartment. Later in the day, your grandma and your godfather will join us and your stepmother and we will mark the occasion by a walk up to Montmartre and the Sacré-Coeur. (Thus affording me the opportunity to demonstrate that the relatively compact dimensions of this city make it an ideal home for someone being pushed everywhere in a wheelchair.) We will have lunch at a café and we will watch the world go by. This will subsequently prompt me to briefly speculate if this is one of the reasons why you look so utterly at home here. Obviously, like many people with your particular range of problems, you spend a certain amount of time every day just watching the world go by so perhaps it makes sense to live somewhere where such a diversion is considered a noble and legitimate pastime!

Vive l'observateur passif!

Isn't this one of the things that Paris is rightly famous for?

After lunch, we will accede to your requests and visit Les Galeries Lafayette and, although on this occasion we will return to the apartment empty handed, we will both be able to take a certain measure of delight every time a reference is made to going 'home'.

In the evening you will have cake and a birthday tea and we will all watch a film together. But there is nothing in the day that lies ahead that will compare to these first few moments as you are waking up. It is something I will cherish for the rest of my life. I go over to the window and open the shutters. It is a beautiful spring morning and the sunlight pours into your room. It illuminates your smiling face lying on the pillow and looking up at me. Then, something else catches my eye. On your mantelpiece, acting as the grand centrepiece beneath your mirror, there is the wooden scale model of a sailing ship that you were given as a Christmas present. It is a magnificent item about two feet from stem to stern. On the prow of the boat there is now a little silver name-plate that I had made a couple of weeks ago. It says WISHBOAT and here in your room your ship will rest for the time being until the day comes for us to sail it somewhere else. Who knows when that will be or what destination will be chosen but every day we're in Paris you can wake up and be comforted by the consolations of possibility and opportunity. In the meantime it sits there as a little icon, a metaphor and a reminder to us both.

I say happy birthday to you and through your Paris window on a fine April morning I feel that a new season is beginning and, as a consequence, I realise one is surely passing.

Third Season

Too Full Of Heaven

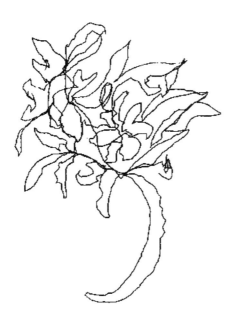

You are one year and 183 days old and I confess that I am having a really bad day. It happens from time to time, no particular cause or reason, just that unmistakable sensation of it all getting on top of me.

I would be the first to admit that I have been feeling a bit depressed recently. Nothing major or clinical, nothing even particularly defined, it is not even something worth articulating or burdening friends with. It's just one of those periodic descents into doom and damnation. Suddenly it is a world without hope and beauty and, while I tell myself it has nothing to do with you or your condition, the fact remains that you are 18 months old and have still shown no signs of any real development.

The past few months have not passed entirely without incident; for example, there is an incident almost every time we revisit the hospital! Since the information became public that there is a claim being made on your behalf, there is a detectable shift in the attitude we regularly encounter from some of the staff there. At best, we experience a sort of lofty derision, at worst, a downright hostility. It's not a particularly pleasant environment and one that I am usually keen to leave.

But the more time passes, the more I am forced to confront the fact that there has been little change or any real progress to speak of. No faltering first steps, no crawling, no attempts at standing, no babbling (beyond that one notable occasion last Christmas), no reaching for things, no tracking your hands. Not one single landmark in 'standard' development and there are to this day still a few lingering doubts about your hearing. In the meantime I have discovered nothing glaringly obvious I can present to doctors and specialists that reinforces my belief in you.

I admit that *sometimes* it all gets a bit desperate.

You lie on the floor next to me while I eat my lunch and you stare into space and today I picture the two of us aged 50 and 20, then 60 and 30, 70 and 40 in exactly the same position with me talking away to you and you just lying there. At that moment all hope freezes.

For one of the few times in our lives together, I recognise the wretched alternative, the other version, their version, I acknowledge the big *what if*...

With some effort, I force myself to abandon this train of thought and to cheer us both up I make up a little story and tell it to you while you are having your tea. It is a story all about a little girl called Sophie.

Sophie was so beautiful and wise and so full of love and brilliance and kindness and understanding that there was no room for anything else. She wasn't able to walk or talk or do all the usual boring things.

'She was too full of heaven.'

Sensing, on reflection quite correctly, that perhaps we might both benefit from some time away from our usual routine, the following day I take you up to the Royal Academy to see the Pop Art Retrospective. It is the first time I have actually taken you to an exhibition and it seems that you really enjoy yourself.

It was, I admit, partly a whim but I wondered how you might respond to seeing paintings on a wall as opposed to in a book. We set off for town really early this morning, figuring, not inaccurately as it happens, that the RA might possibly be less crowded at that time of the day. I choose the buggy over the sling and this transpires to be the sensible choice.

I push you around the galleries, stopping in front of any painting that seems to catch your interest. Whether it is the scale of the work or the subject matter that appeals to you I have no idea but you seem totally absorbed by what you are looking at. I have never seen you so engrossed by anything in your short life.

86

Personally, I'm not sure if it is actually possible to actively like Pop Art any more than it is possible to actively dislike it. I went to the exhibition with no particular opinion and came away equally indifferent. The most powerful sensation being the odd blast of nostalgia, which seems entirely inappropriate. A simple longing for good old-fashioned (pre-post) modernism perhaps?

We stay there for an hour or so during which time you definitely display a leaning towards the more abstract paintings, early Hockney, Larry Rivers and Kitaj rather than Rosenquist and Warhol. You gaze at these with a sort of beatific expression on your face and I feel that we have made an important discovery of some kind this morning.

You get a bit stiff after a while and with some regret I decide that it's time for us to make tracks for home.

On the way back, taking advantage of your moral support, we call in to see my editor. I grovel quite shamelessly for ten minutes and then apologise for the last piece being so late and for the couple of features I had to turn down in the summer because you had chicken pox. He doesn't seem too bothered although something tells me that this might not be the best time to ask for money.

The conversation then shifts on to the subject of a new magazine that is in the pipeline and he asks me if I fancy doing a little sub-editing for a couple of months, 'just while it gets off the ground'.

But I look at you and you don't seem all that impressed either.

I say no.

Then suddenly I'm thinking I'm sick of being paid late, I'm sick of chasing around the place, I'm sick of deadlines hanging over me when you aren't well and I'm especially sick of labouring over articles no one will ever read for magazines no one has ever heard of.

I'm worn out, I tell him, and I want a rest from it.

We leave the matter with me 'taking a break' for a couple of months but I have no intention of writing any more features for him or anyone else for that matter. You have to come first now and that bout of chicken pox brought everything home to me. I can't guarantee anyone anything; you have to be number one nowadays.

We return home and rather than consider what has just occurred as my retirement, I do my very best to feel suitably liberated.

You are one year and 262 days old and after weeks and months of planning and anticipation, I take you in a cab to our local day centre for pre-school children with disabilities. Recently built, it's called something else, something much grander and infinitely less specific but I fear I instantly forget the name upon being told it. We have gone there partly to have a bit of a look around as you might one day be offered a place there but mainly we are there to meet the music therapy department.

I get you dressed up in your best new clothes and you really do look particularly beautiful today.

The centre is impressive, I must say. Very well equipped and laid out and the staff seem very friendly and efficient.

We meet the music therapists, two ladies about my age, and we chat about you and the role that music therapy will hopefully play in your development. We then talk about the importance of music generally and I make the mistake of mentioning Iggy Pop, for which I receive a couple of fiercely blank stares.

Suitably embarrassed, I feel less inclined thereafter to say anything.

Music therapy still sounds a little vague to me but at the very least I have now stopped thinking about children in vests and pants running around roughly in time to the *Carnival of the Animals*. Yes, things have changed a lot since I was a child.

But we shall see when you have your first 'session' in a couple of weeks.

I say goodbye and I am making my way back to the main entrance when it happens.

Another moment in the endless chain of moments I have been dreading.

As we pass through the main open-plan area, the children are brought over to say goodbye to us. Half a dozen or so little boys and girls, some with cerebral palsy, some with Down's Syndrome. Others have problems that are not immediately obvious: one little boy is deaf and blind but each little boy and each little girl, in his or her own way, is *extraordinary*.

All have stories like yours, some are probably worse, all have seen that anguished look, that fear in the eyes of their parents. All of them have a history, all of them are survivors. Then it hits me and suddenly I can see another version of you, *their* version, another classification, another category – another one that I stubbornly refuse to acknowledge.

These are your peers, you are now one among many. These are the people against whom your progress will be charted and measured. You are amongst those who will now and forever be regarded as your people. This is your world and you will, in time, learn to dream your dreams within these parameters.

As I will have to learn to dream mine.

Suddenly, I feel that I have to leave the place.

I quickly tell everyone that we have to go outside and wait for our cab. I just about manage to get us through the door as the tears start running down my face.

The following morning I spend writing on my computer with you sitting on my lap. At the end of my endeavours, I turn your head towards the screen, as I always do, and read passages out to you. I move the cursor around the screen and try to get you to follow what I am reading. It might be a case of wishful thinking but you seem to enjoy this part of our daily routine. You smile at me and in a small way it blocks out some of the memory of yesterday. I save the file, which is actually the prologue to a possible novel, but prefer not to think of it in such Big Terms.

I feel quite pleased with what I've written but as a character nearly said today: *We tend to judge ourselves simply as successes or failures. But the reality is that usually we are neither.*

A couple of weeks later I take you to your first music therapy appointment and I am allowed to observe the session at a discreet distance. The session is unlike anything I could have ever imagined and I actually find it a rather humbling experience. I watch in a stunned silence as the most extraordinary half an hour plays itself out in front of me.

Firstly, I hear you making noises in the back of your throat and changing pitch with the piano, not the most musically edifying sound in the world but enough for the therapist to assure me at the end of the session that you can certainly hear well enough. If you never do anything else in music therapy then that on its own was certainly worth waiting for.

But there is more. At the end of the session you are sat at the piano and after a tremendous effort and with all the concentration you can muster you manage to hit the keys with your fist! Just the once but it was enough.

I come away feeling elated and feel certain that somewhere locked away, deep down inside you, a part of you is feeling pretty elated too.

The second and third sessions are no less remarkable but sadly we have to postpone the fourth because we have to travel to Manchester for an appointment with an 'expert' paediatrician. Your solicitor has been keen to state the importance of seeing experts based as far away from London as possible. It rules out any possibility of 'professional conflict'.

It is a gruelling and exhausting day and you are forced to spend eight hours on a train. By the time we finally meet the expert, you are hardly at your best.

And neither am I.

He asks me about your progress and as usual I try to stress all the positive things. In doing so I am quite aware that I'm in danger of sounding like I'm canvassing support on behalf of music therapy. He smiles and nods his head a bit in the traditional manner but I know he isn't paying the slightest attention to me. I am, by this stage, thoroughly worn out by the day and feel a great surge of anger rise up in me.

I want to jump on to his desk and shout at him. Tell him that I know exactly what he is thinking, that I know perfectly well what is going through his mind. But he is completely wrong. COMPLETELY WRONG! Understand? And no, I am not in denial, I am quite the opposite!

Yes, I want to scream at him, I took you to the RA to see the Pop Art show, why not? I am not saying you fully understood it or appreciated it. But guess what? That wasn't the point! When we stood looking at all those great paintings together, we shared the experience and we were equals. Just for once we were not able-bodied or disabled, but simply EQUALS! I happen to be very proud of you and I didn't want you being forced to stay at home!

PROUD?

(Oh what fresh denial is this?)

First the disbelief then the pity.

But they miss the point. Always, they miss the point!

I will continue in this way not because I refuse to accept 'the problems'. I will do so precisely because I am completely aware of 'the problems'.

It's quite simple, really.

Pity no one ever thought of it.

But of course, I say nothing. I just thank him for his time. Then we chat about Manchester for a while and I yearn for the safe, good, placid, kind train that will take us away from it.

*   *   *

91

You are two years old today and the day is celebrated in the usual manner, although from a personal angle I wonder if I wouldn't actually prefer to celebrate the day that you finally left hospital – June the whatever it was. That seems a greater source of joy and fonder memories. Anyway, this year at least you seem to show an *understanding* that this is your special day and if I wasn't so scared of sounding like a deluded father, I might be tempted to comment on the fact that you seem to be relishing the attention. You certainly appeared to enjoy being helped to unwrap your presents.

At 5.30, I leave you having a cuddle from your grandma and sneak away for a few minutes' solitude. I seem to do this without really thinking, like I was following some latent biological urge. Alone, I reflect back and back and back to that minute point in time, that tiny dot in infinity. That moment after which...

I stop myself.

But this year, I think, a light has been switched on somewhere. It is only a flickering ten watts or so but compared to the great darkness that preceded it, sometimes I swear it glows brighter than a million suns.

You are twelve years and 41 days old and today, as well as being a resident of Paris, you become a resident of the fine old city of Canterbury. Well, to be entirely accurate, we have moved to a small, quite pretty village about three miles away but for the purposes of postcodes and council taxes, we are now considered residents of Canterbury.

This has not been the easiest of moves and by comparison the relocation to Paris was infinitely simpler. This is partly a result of the difference in conveyancing practices and attitudes in the two countries and partly the result of fate and bad luck. But finally we are here and the long process of selling and buying is over and we can enjoy the rest of our summer.

Another small landmark is passed earlier today and we are now officially living with your stepmother, stepsister and stepbrother. We all choose to mark the occasion by spending the greater part of the day with you, unpacking all the crates and boxes that boast the legend:

SOPHIE – bedroom!!

It is a long process and over the hours, in an attempt to absorb the general tedium, I start to reflect for the first time on those items you decided to send to Paris all those months ago and those you have selected to remain in England. After the most fleeting deliberation, it becomes quite evident that you have been following a very strict idea about what you feel is right for each location. I find it absolutely fascinating that you have two such very distinct projections of yourself. Paris definitely seems to reflect your more artistic side, with everything roughly connected to painting and music, as well as most of your pictures and books being packed off there. Your room in Paris is now busy and cluttered with art and cushions like the abode of any self-respecting twelve-year-old bohemian.

By contrast, an old property in the English countryside evidently inspires in you a set of very different ideas. All the items we have been unpacking today and your choice of décor and colour for your room seem to conform to some fairly strict notion of being genteel and feminine. The walls are mostly blank and free from decoration and the whole vibe seems to be one of calm and understatement, which is such a contrast to Paris. I suppose it's a fairly simple means by which you demonstrate that you are no longer a child and that you are no longer to be treated as such. Personally, I am always delighted when you exhibit such strong ideas about aspects of your own life and make decisions with such an extraordinary clarity of purpose.

I confess I have been so wrapped up with both the moves of late and the whole notion of dividing our time between two countries, such a major step in both our lives in so many respects, that I'd not really considered the possible virtues of alternating a very urban environment with a much more tranquil and rural one. This naturally gives you access to all manner of different experiences.

Actually, it is your new GP who first points this out to me as we go along to register later in our first week. He tells you that you are lucky to have the best of both worlds and I claim once again on behalf of intent and design that which would be more fairly attributed to accident or luck.

He also raises with me the question of schools and I explain that I've already had a number of meetings with our local education authority with a view to finding an appropriate school or schools for the start of the new term. In fact, after some consideration, it would now appear that the best method of providing you with a suitable education would be to divide your school time three ways: between a mainstream comprehensive school, a special school and home tuition. In principle this seems like a very sensible and eminently practical solution.

The mainstream school, your attendance at which I privately consider to be your supreme scholastic achievement, will give you the mental stimulation you will need, while the special school will keep you in contact with all the specialists and therapists. The home tuition will, I imagine, continue with the now well-established methods and also back up your academic work. I tell him that I have been assured that there shouldn't be a problem with this particular combination and, after all, your Statement of Special Educational Needs, which has been hammered out in blood and tears (mostly mine) over the last few years, is particularly specific about that sort of thing. The GP smiles and wishes us luck and I think no more about it.

For the next few weeks we busy ourselves leisurely exploring our new locality. Our fellow villagers and all manner of ducks and horses seem reasonably cordial towards us and it is a very agreeable way to spend a lazy summer. At the end of our road, no more than 200 yards from our front door, there is a little wood that runs down to a river. Remarkably, we have found a little route by which we can navigate your wheelchair through the trees as far as the riverbank. I take you down there most afternoons just for an hour or so and I have to concede that you do manage to look terribly at home in such an environment.

I point out to you this afternoon that the only sartorial quirk that you are missing for these afternoon trips is a floppy summer hat of some description, but sadly you have judged your summer head wear to be 'arty' rather than 'lady' and so they are all in France! Then, just in time, I realise that I'm about to stumble headlong into one of those traditional *Oh, of course, you know* all *about it now* parent and teenager speeches and I manage to stop myself. It's a nice day and I don't think either of us is quite ready for something of that magnitude.

I enjoy these weeks that we spend in this unhurried manner but I am aware that this doesn't signify a conclusion but merely a respite. If I have learned anything over the past twelve years it is simply that our story modifies, adapts and even alters beyond all recognition but it continues.

And so it continues.

Its basic themes, I have lately come to realise, remain fixed and constant and so I simply regard these weeks as a welcome break from the usual.

Then, as we approach the beginning of the new term and there has been no further communication or news on the subject of your school, I confess that I begin to wonder. I look back over our recent weeks and sympathise with Larkin's line somewhere in which he refers to an imagined golden summer of 1913. 'After which it was not the same.'

As we pass the first week in September and there is still no news, I begin to make phone calls. There are a few problems, I'm told, but they promise that they will get back to me. This does not bode well and I put the phone down in particularly low spirits. Meanwhile, the weekend is upon us and your godmother, who has recently qualified as a teacher and who stood in as your home tutor a couple of times earlier in the year, comes down to stay for a few days. She is in the process of separating from her husband and is desperately wanting to move out of London. She is very taken with the village and tonight, as I settle you off to sleep, I am sure that I can hear, over the owls and the distant seagulls, the great heavenly wheels of coincidence once again rotating in your favour.

You are twelve years and 173 days old and I receive the phone call that I have been dreading, yet half-expecting. It seems that it has not been possible to offer you a place at the mainstream comprehensive. Not even for a day or a couple of lessons each week. This decision has been taken, or so the school claims, because of a lack of suitable wheelchair access but I must admit I'm not convinced.

This is a real blow to our plans and I take the news badly, passing through fury and anger before settling into a sort of shrugging, muted cynicism. As though I have been utterly naïve to have expected things to be any different. At least, I suppose there is some comfort to be gained in the feeling that we're back on familiar ground once again.

Besides, I tell you after I have broken the news, the school in question is named after a saint and I went to a school named after a saint too and very rarely in my experience do such places justify the sanctity of their nomenclature.

I make a few phone calls and complain about the situation but slowly I surrender myself to the general futility of it all. It makes very little difference if it's a question of policy, principle or personality. Or if the issue is local or national. As has happened so many times in the past, it really doesn't matter why this problem has arisen, and looking for underlying reasons or routes by which I can apportion blame or responsibility is time consuming and ultimately pointless. Worse than that it is an unforgivable waste of your time too and it doesn't move you even fractionally nearer your goal. The man said 'accreditation', didn't he? I realise now that somewhere there is a clock that has just started ticking.

While we sit and wait for an alternative to present itself and, as we are now lacking the routine of the school day, I take advantage of the opportunity and we spend some more time in Paris together. We are getting quite accustomed to our trips nowadays yet, despite this, I do notice a certain euphoric expression on your face whenever we disembark at the Gare du Nord. Invariably, the first person we see when we arrive at our apartment is Jean, the concierge's son. Therefore, the first thing I usually say in Paris is *'Bonjour, Jean,'* which is also, rather tragically, the first thing that most people of my age ever learned in a French lesson. So much for progress! But, I tell myself, there can be found in this simple act an enjoyable symmetry.

Having exhausted so many of the major attractions in the past, we now occupy our days visiting a number of alternative tourist spots: Picasso's studio in Montmartre, the house where Van Gogh used to stay, Serge Gainsbourg's house on the Left Bank and anything else I can think of. We go for long walks and attempt to make the most of your truancy.

Meanwhile I do a lot of thinking.

We are not long into our visit before I start to acknowledge the familiarity of the general situation regarding your education in England. That depressing yet recognisable sensation of having achieved so much coupled with the realisation that we are going to have to start all over again. All the great work of the past few years, all the amazing things that you've done will, I realise, count for very little. The move away from London is basically a return to the starting point. As has happened so many times before, we are going to have to rely on our own endeavours to move things along. I thought my job was done, I was wrong. Please forgive me.

97

We go for a stroll one morning up to the Sacré-Coeur and we look out at the whole of Paris stretched out before us. This is a good place to make promises to you, I think, and so I make one. I tell you that I will sort out your education and I will do whatever it takes to ensure that one day you will get all the credit and respect you deserve. I promise you that I will do everything I can to achieve this and I'm not going to sit around any longer and wait for things to sort themselves out.

It makes a sort of sense that if you require anything even slightly unorthodox then you shouldn't be wasting your time with established orthodoxies. You should transcend their petty limitations as soon as possible. Feeling suitably defiant, I let Paris be my witness and I tell you that even very small revolutions have to start somewhere.

Ours can start here.

You are 2 years and 32 days old and I take you to your regular music therapy session. You are a little under the weather today and the whole venture is a waste of time really. You are tired and unresponsive so I have a chat to the therapists while you briefly doze in your buggy.

It seems that the powers that be are threatening to close down the music therapy department; apparently it was only an experiment or something. They need all the help and support they can get. I offer to write a letter on their behalf, which is the very least I can do.

Finally, you have a means by which we can observe and monitor your development (all the sessions are video recorded) and after a couple of months, just long enough to become fully dependent on the service, they try and take it away from us.

Brilliant!

I go home and immediately start composing a letter.

In the meantime, I am given a very positive angle on your development a week or so later from a hugely improbable source.

God, it would seem, continues to employ the most unlikely messengers.

I have taken you to Guy's Hospital to see a dentist, who specialises in treating children with disabilities. Your teeth are in poor condition I learn today due to the high sugar content in the soya milk you were drinking for your first 12 months. I must confess I have not over-burdened myself in the past with concern about your teeth but I promise to be more vigilant in future. Anyway, as you and I are waiting to see the dentist, I chat to the assistant.

She looks into your mouth and asks me if you ever grind your teeth. Constantly, I tell her, fearing that this might be contributing to their poor state of repair. She smiles and tells me that in her experience, children with your history who grind their teeth do so out of frustration.

She clarifies this by confirming what I suspected; that a child showing frustration is showing an awareness. Before frustration comes expectation, she adds, and one could take all this as a very positive sign.

She restates that this was only in *her* experience and only a simple observation but I fear I have stopped listening again. You and I are off once more, floating off and away, over London Bridge Station, circling the City and St Paul's before disappearing over the horizon in a great explosion of rainbows.

Over the next few weeks, you are visited regularly at home by your new physiotherapist. On one occasion she brings with her a woman who she introduces as a speech therapist. Both exhibit a very positive and open-minded attitude, which I find particularly refreshing. I also detect a certain delightful irreverence in their manner, which is obviously genuine and quite spontaneous.

They both ask me what I 'feel' about your perception and general awareness of things and both refer to the importance of intuition in dealing with children with 'profound' difficulties. This seems such a refreshing change from the norm that I almost feel like crying.

I am interested in speech therapy and I learn today that you are officially classed as 'non-verbal'. Then I make the mistake that I have been making all my life since I asked my father at the age of four why birds flew. In answer to that particular enquiry, my father – ever the pragmatist, ever the man of science – drew me a diagram on a piece of paper, explained air currents and aerodynamics to me and basically *how* birds flew. I thanked him, having not understood a single word, and went away as baffled as ever. There was of course an important lesson to be learned there but sadly I have chosen to ignore it for over a quarter of a century. This afternoon, I ask about the mechanics of speech and am presented with a lengthy air currents and aerodynamics answer.

Back on safer ground, I am shown how to sit you on my lap, particularly if we are sitting at the computer for more than a couple of minutes. This I learn is good 'postural management' and prevents you from going too stiff, into 'extension'.

When they leave, I sit you on my lap in the prescribed fashion and we write another couple of hundred words together.

The following week, as if I needed a stark contrast to our afternoon with the speech therapist, I finally get to see a copy of the report on you from the paediatrician in Manchester. It is the most damning document I have ever seen. Every other line seems to feature prominently the words 'she will never...'

All day I torture myself with these words and by the evening I think I know whole sections of the report off by heart.

Is this the price of justice?

Or is this simply one of those days about which your solicitor warned me two years ago, a day when I have to keep reminding myself that *it is all for you?*

The following days I spend under a cloud that doesn't lift until I take you to the day centre for your music therapy. We are greeted with the good news that the department has won its fight and will remain where it is at least for the time being, which hopefully will take care of your needs until you are in school full-time. I am thanked for my letter and I am delighted to have played an active part, however small.

I chat to the music therapists at the end of your session while your physiotherapist and her assistant whisk you away to do some brief exercises with you in another part of the building. When I collect you I am told that they have been playing a game with you.

They ask me if I have ever observed you blinking in a particular slow and deliberate manner. I say that I have done and had actually wondered if this might have been something to do with you being long-sighted (this is not as naïve as it sounds – a friend does exactly the same thing and blames it on his long-sightedness.) But I am wrong about this in your case.

Your slow, deliberate blinking, I am assured, is a 'Yes' response.

It is your way of answering in the affirmative to a question and not an uncommon response in 'non-verbal' children. One explanation, and the one that makes the most sense to me, is that when we nod our heads in response to questions we often simultaneously lower our eyelids for a brief moment or two. Children with your particular range of problems observe this over time and being unable to nod their heads in the conventional way develop this 'yes response' as a method of suggesting or implying a nod.

I am totally taken aback by all this.

But they demonstrate the method effectively by asking you simple questions and I observe your responses. Do you like music? ('Yes.') Did you like your dinner today? (No response.) And so on. My head reels with the possibilities, while your physiotherapist and her assistant continue with the questions.

They talk about the possible applications.

As ever, I would much rather talk about the possible implications.

After a couple of weeks of using this 'yes' response, I realise that a whole new world has been unlocked. Sometimes I am so focused on trying to prove your intelligence in the long-term, I fear I lose sight of all the practical day-to-day possibilities. There I was thinking this might be a valid means of confirming that you definitely process information and that you are showing an appropriate level of understanding, yet I failed to see immediately what a true gift it was.

You can now, in the most basic way, communicate your needs and it is even possible to have what might best be described as 'binary conversations' with you. Provided the questions continue to be yes/no choices, the exchange can become more detailed and, from your point of view, more specific.

Do you want lunch now?

Would you like something hot?

Would you like chicken? And so on.

It takes practice but the rewards are fantastic. You can make your own decisions and express your opinions.

This afternoon I ask you if you would like to sit on my lap while I do some more to chapter six. 'Yes.' Shall I read this new bit out to you? 'Yes.'

Like I say, the rewards are fantastic.

I show off your new talents when we are visited at home the following week by the consultant paediatrician from Guy's. On the whole the appointment is encouraging and the general tone positive.

One of the topics she raises is quite new to me. She asks me if you have a sense of humour. Do you laugh in context? When you do laugh, I tell her, yes, it is usually in context.

She explains that this whole area interests her a great deal as it is one of the most overlooked aspects of child development. Even the most basic comedy, perhaps the slapstick of circus clowns, functions within a framework of previously assimilated information. A flower that squirts water is only 'funny' because we know what a flower is and we know it doesn't do that.

Humour in this context requires learning.

Thus a child who laughs appropriately is exhibiting knowledge and an awareness of context. A banana is not funny *per se*, but taken out of context and stuck in someone's ear it becomes a comic device. Well, it does if you're two.

I find all this quite fascinating and wonder if I will live long enough to see comedy therapy taking its place on the curriculum.

All those kids with special needs being assessed by their capacity to laugh.

Now that would be a development!

You are two years and 267 days old and you have your first full day at the day centre. While you are there I make the trip into town to see our solicitor. We discuss developments in some detail and go over the reports that have already been assembled. It has troubled me that these experts are so single-minded in their appraisals. Now, I realise that for the purposes of the trial everything must be based around the legal version of you, a version that focuses only on particular selected facets. This version takes its place alongside the medical and educational versions.

There is a true you of course, a complex and enigmatic person and a version far greater than the sum of all the others. But still I feel that sometimes this complete version remains invisible to everyone except me.

I return home in low spirits and receive a phone call from one of your therapists informing me that she is leaving next week and would like to call in to say goodbye. She visits the following day and I'll be sorry to see the back of her. She has always been very understanding and positive in her outlook – one of 'Us' in other words. As she is leaving, she turns to me and says, 'You know, I think that one day you'll find out that Sophie's problems are about ninety per cent *physical*. I am sure everything else will be fine.'

I would be tempted to dismiss this as little more than a parting off-the-record nicety if it wasn't for the absolute conviction with which she spoke. Whether she is right or wrong, she certainly believed what she said. I thank her and wish her all the best.

Hard to explain how I feel, maybe more vindicated than elated. It is a small step, a tiny signpost, meaningless to everyone but to me it represents a start.

The following week is an impossibly busy one for you and never have so many versions of you been on display in such a short time.

On Monday we are visited at home by an 'expert' physiotherapist sent by our solicitor. Then in the afternoon I take you to Guy's for another dental appointment and you escape with a couple of fillings. Then on Tuesday morning we have a visit from a paediatric neurologist sent by The Other Side. Despite my fears, to my utter surprise, the man was absolutely charming. He examines you thoroughly and we talk about your development. That is the development of the legal version naturally. He actually seemed to go along with the 'mainly physical' prognosis and I may have relished such a confirmation had I not had to drag you (medical version) off to Guy's so you could be cast for your spinal brace.

This device (termed a 'jacket'), which resembles a thick plastic corset moulded to the exact contours of your body, is to be worn for initially six hours a day. Its purpose is to keep the spine as straight as possible and thus prevent all manner of problems later on.

Your brace, they tell me, will be the smallest one that has ever been made at Guy's.

The week concludes with my appointment with your music therapists during which we discuss the projected meeting next week of all the therapists at the day centre. Your progress and the plans for the future will be discussed at this meeting and a lot of the points I want to make involve music therapy. The videos of your sessions are obviously really important and today we go through a few edited bits, picking out the best

104

examples. I realise that this might be the closest I have come to tangible proof of your cognitive functioning. I am nervous about this meeting, *very* nervous in fact, and I return home exhausted and notice that I have developed a twitch around my left temple.

I am not in the least surprised.

Finally, the day of the meeting dawns; such things are officially termed, I learn today, Multi-Disciplinary Meetings, an expression that conjures up all manner of images, none of which I would wish to dwell on particularly. I sit amongst half a dozen therapists for a couple of hours reviewing reports and observations and planning strategies for the immediate future. The idea behind these meetings is that all the 'services' are co-ordinated and all decisions are made by 'the team' and not by individuals. In principle it seems like a very sound idea.

The 'yes response' is discussed; a few doubts, as I could have probably anticipated, are raised as 'the observations have been inconsistent'. The subject of abnormal movements is discussed and they will monitor more carefully all the twitches and spasms they observe.

By this point in the meeting I must confess I am a little restless – I want to grab you and rush out of the door again. (Will I ever grow out of this impulse? Probably not, I fear.) But it is only the medical/educational versions under discussion, I tell myself.

At the climax of the meeting it is time to reveal a new version, the musical version!

The music therapist sets up the video and talks us through half a dozen examples of your work this past year. It is by any standards an impressive archive and I'm sure I detect some of the less positive mouths in the room dropping open at certain points.

To reinforce this, at the end of the meeting I try to make the point that if you *can't* reach for things or track objects, etc. in orthodox surroundings but you do so in music therapy, then we must be a little more careful about using the word 'can't'. Should we perhaps look more carefully at the method of stimulation?

I conclude by saying that we should all work from an understanding of what you *can* do rather than concentrating on what you can't.

You are three years old today and we pass another small landmark. As the day coincides with one of your days at the day centre, they arrange a party for you there. Your first birthday away from home and you seem to enjoy every minute of it. While you are there I rush around getting last-minute presents for you – thankfully, the more your character develops, the easier you are to buy presents for.

The development of personality in your case seems to have coincided with the development of hair follicles and now, looking back at photos taken this time last year, I can see just how much your hair has grown. It is thick and curly now and falls in ringlets around your face.

You are more beautiful than ever.

But not a superficial beauty, not a surface beauty; a great deep Dionysian beauty. Not fleeting or transitory but truly eternal. A spiritual beauty that, denied a means of expression, somehow exudes from every atom of your being.

I love you more than I thought it was actually possible to love another human being. The fact that sometimes you seem to be aware of this is the source of the very greatest joy imaginable.

Happy birthday, daughter.

The following few weeks are mainly quiet ones and pass without incident apart from the afternoon we go for a look around the assessment centre that you will start attending shortly. Prior to the drafting of a Statement of Special Educational Needs, children attend a centre like this where their strengths and abilities can be monitored. After which a place will be allocated at an appropriate school. Naturally, as this now brings you under the auspices of the Department of Education, the place, from the outside at least, looks like a fairly ordinary primary school.

I must confess that I do not fall in love with the place. After your day centre, it has an antiseptic *municipality* about it. I find it all a little grim. I meet the staff, and whilst some are extremely clued-up, others look a little worn down by it all. One of the classroom helpers actually asks me how I cope!

It was one of those afternoons.

However, I try to put it all out of my mind and concentrate on other things. Luckily there are a couple of available distractions. For example, we take a trip up to Guy's where we are now finally able to collect your body brace. I gaze at the finished item in a kind of bemused wonder. A thick plastic corset that fastens around the front with a couple of thick leather straps. There are two attachments, which fit around the top of your legs to keep your hips in the proper position. I confess that it's a bit of a shock seeing you in it for the first time but not nearly as horrific as I had been anticipating.

It is obviously beneficial in preventing any further spinal problems and I must say that you tolerate it reasonably well. The brace gives you a rigid, fixed posture with a straight, stiff back and torso. Your head control is still a little erratic, however, and the resulting effect when you are sitting on my lap I find oddly reminiscent of Alison Steadman's character in *Abigail's Party* for some reason.

You are three years and 164 days old. We near the end of your time at your day centre and prepare ourselves for the move to the assessment centre, a move that will ultimately involve you going to the school on the 'special bus'. I find all this rather depressing, I must say.

I take you to your music therapy session this morning and learn from the therapist that your sessions will cease when you leave the day centre. The assessment centre comes under Education whereas the day centre is Health.

I am stunned by this.

Suddenly there is this great sense of 'They' again. 'They' can't do this to 'Us'. Surely it isn't fair that 'They' are *allowed* to do this to 'Us'. In my rage and confusion I do something which I quickly regret, I start complaining to your music therapist in a manner that might have been a little more volatile than the situation warranted. I ask her how she could let this happen to you but I know I am directing my anger at the wrong person.

She is not the problem, of course.

She is on our side, she is one of 'Us'.

I speak to the music therapist again on the phone later on in the afternoon and apologise for my outburst. I ask her if there is anything I can do to improve the situation. In short, you have to go to this assessment centre and thus you will lose your music therapy. The only advice she offers is that I try approaching the Director of Education.

Firstly, however, I do something that I never could have pictured myself doing. I write a long impassioned letter to my MP.

In essence I ask a simple question. How can you be provided with this one single marvellous opportunity of expressing yourself, of learning and of understanding – the best means we have of assessing your intelligence and abilities – and then just have it taken away from you? As I loudly trumpet at the conclusion of my letter, 'by any moral standpoint you might care to mention, it is unjust and unethical.'

I go for a stroll late in the evening and post it.

For once in my life I feel that I am ranting appropriately.

The following day I write two more letters on behalf of music therapy, trying to drum up support and generally complaining about the situation. I have heard for the past three years how this system caters for the child's individual needs. The word 'individual' is misleading, perhaps they should use 'personal' instead. Everything I have seen suggests the child's needs are catered for provided that they are not *too* individual.

Eventually I find that I am in correspondence with no fewer than six different people about your music therapy (very encouraging 'quotable' letter back from our MP by the way), and have had meetings with more people than I care to remember. I now have a few insights into the workings of the Special Needs system and see very little to cheer about.

Then, totally out of the blue one afternoon the following week, I receive the most extraordinary phone call. Absolutely unbelievable! Somebody high up in the Special Needs section at the Directorate of Education rings me to tell me that there is a 'strong possibility' that they will make an 'exception' and allow you to continue your music therapy under the banner of Education when you transfer to the assessment centre.

You will be the first child ever to have this.

I take all this in but I confess I feel uncomfortable about the implications; I don't like the idea of music therapy being offered to one child because that child's father moaned about it. It still doesn't seem fair. Who is being assessed here? The children or their parents? Exception? I don't like the sound of that. No, I think, I have come this far and suggest that if you are made a *precedent* rather than an exception then I would be happy with that. She can't answer this herself but says she will call back. I hang up, expecting to hear nothing further. I am quite taken aback when she calls about five minutes later.

'Yes,' she says, 'that's been agreed then. Sophie will continue to have her music therapy and if you feel strongly about it then I don't see why we shouldn't view this as a precedent.'

She concludes by stressing that your needs and the needs of children like you constitute 'only a small percentage of a small percentage'.

I thank her and replace the receiver. I let the news sink in and feel a deep sense of satisfaction. I have done something for you and together we have done something for music therapy, which I suppose is the least we can do. Immediately I start to feel as though I am coming down with a cold.

The following week you spend your final day at the day centre. This place has done so much for you and so many of your great achievements have occurred within the confines of these four walls. The staff have all been so supportive and positive during your time here and I take a bouquet of four-dozen red roses for them as a gesture of appreciation to divide amongst themselves.

I know that, sooner or later, we are going to miss this place.

You are twelve years and 254 days old and the New Year has brought with it no sudden great change in fortune and our lives continue in very much the same way as the previous one. There has been no further news about a suitable school placement for you. We have been offered another couple of days at another special school but this feels like a rather desperate token gesture and hardly represents a solution. There has been no action taken whatsoever on my requests to find you another mainstream comprehensive school. Furthermore, my phone calls and e-mails are now frequently going unanswered, which, experience has taught me, is seldom an indication that things are progressing in a positive manner.

Your grandma comes and stays for a couple of days and I welcome the opportunity of her giving you a couple of art lessons. She's been doing this for a couple of years now in her own particular fashion. I should perhaps point out that your grandma is an art teacher or rather she was until she retired a few years ago. She is also a professional artist.

She talks to you about paintings, explains various techniques to you and then puts a pen or a brush in your hand, supports your arm and lets you have a go and experiment. I used to consider it a therapeutic hour or so, or at the very least a bit of fun and some special time you could share with your grandma. Nowadays, however, it counts as very welcome stimulation and I am delighted to observe from the sidelines for a few hours.

Deprived of school and other means of expression, you seem to be devoting a lot of your energy to your painting at the moment. I've always known that you had a great love of art, ever since I took you to that Pop Art show when you were about 18 months old. You have always adored Picasso and I can remember being able to soothe the agonies of your teething by showing you a book of Picasso's paintings. Nothing else, as I recall, had anything like the calming influence of those pictures. Later on, you fell under the spell of Matisse, Klee, Kandinsky, Miro, Rothko, Jackson Pollock and a whole host of others, but Picasso still retains his special place in your heart.

But nowadays I discover that I am observing something else.

This afternoon I watch you and witness a remarkable change taking place. It is subtle at first but unmistakable. Under your grandma's scrutiny, I can see that you are now starting to draw and paint with far greater determination and concentration than I have ever observed in the past. You have always dabbled and doodled and taken great pleasure in the *experience* of painting but this is now developing into something far more focused, far more intense. Anyone observing you could see that this is something that you really desperately want to do. It is a slow process but the sheer will-power you demonstrate and the incredible amount of effort involved ensures that not a moment is wasted. I have rarely seen you work so hard over a couple of hours and yet you seem to be enjoying yourself and the whole process of expression.

Today you are painting a landscape, it is actually the scene by the river where we go to see the horses. It is a bold, assured and confident interpretation and I'm astonished by the finished work, as I have been by a couple of your other pictures in recent weeks. Ever the proud father, as soon as it is dry I put

111

it in a frame and, with your permission, hang it on the wall of my office.

The truth is that you have been improving and developing your own very individual style over these school-less weeks and months during your grandma's regular visits. There is nowadays a very identifiable quality to your work, something tangible that I can recognise in all your paintings and sketches. There is a certain confident economy of line in the drawing and everything seems to be organised and planned very carefully in advance. It is my understanding that you are gradually evolving a method by which you can work within the restrictions of your limited movement.

But it does take it out of you and at the end of each art session you are exhausted.

With some justification, you are quite proud of your paintings and your first question the following day is invariably, 'you like my painting?' I will naturally and quite candidly answer in the affirmative and then enquire if you are also happy with the finished work. You will consider the question for a moment and then almost always proffer the same answer.

'a bit.'

Ever the perfectionist.

Typical artist.

I confess that over recent years I have been too wrapped up in your academic achievements to pay much attention to your artistic leanings.

Mea culpa, daughter!

I knew that painting was something you enjoyed but I wasn't aware that you had been developing such an aptitude for it. I suppose on many levels, it's another means of communication, another way by which you can express yourself. But that makes me sound too much like a therapist. As your father, I think that you are producing some remarkable paintings at the moment and are starting to show a real flair and talent.

Meanwhile a few more weeks slip by and I am still no nearer

sorting out a school for you. During this time your recently single godmother starts house hunting in our village and we put up her and her family while she does so. This allows you to spend some time with her two teenage sons and you watch films and listen to music together. The three of you share some common interests in music and on one occasion, showing yourselves to be kindred spirits of social conscience, you evoke the spirits of Woody Guthrie and Joe Strummer and spend a couple of afternoons writing a protest song together.

Eventually, your godmother finally finds herself a suitable property about half a mile down the road at the other end of the village. Shortly afterwards, she tells me that she is about to start looking for a permanent teaching job in Kent. At this point there forms in my head two very clear, very distinct, yet related questions.

I need answers to both as soon as possible.

And so in pursuit of a quick answer to the first, I make a phone call the following day to your solicitor. I leap straight in with another variation on my most frequently voiced request and I ask him if any more funds could be made available to put towards your education. Before he can answer this initial enquiry and with almost no subtlety whatsoever I lapse into a detailed elaboration in first person plural. Of course, this is a fairly obvious attempt to manipulate proceedings, suggesting that he and I are part of a well-established team working together for your benefit. I probably sound like some frantic door-to-door salesman as I gush hopelessly in such hurried tones that WE are having a few problems sorting out your education and there are serious doubts that WE will be able to find a school for you. And WE really need to sort out a new tutor very soon as WE have already lost so much time.

After a short pause, enough to conclude that my cunning strategy has been all but worthless, he explains that your money is intended to secure, above everything else, your quality of life. To this ultimate end, and within reason, funds can usually be made available. I'm not sure if this has actually answered my question so I put it to him that I would value your education at this point in your life above many other concerns and he agrees with me. Then he asks me what I actually want and I tell him I want the extra money so I can employ a tutor for three days a week.

By his reaction, it appears that my question was precisely the one he was anticipating. He tells me that I am not the only person in this situation and taking such an action is not an uncommon one. He informs me that he can't see there being any objections to this and so he suggests that we try it for a couple of months.

My first question now has a small red tick next to it.

You are twelve years and 273 days old and it is the weekend I get around to asking my second question.

The weekend in question was to have been one of your weekends for staying with your mother. Until recently she was seeing you every other weekend; following to the letter the arrangements that were made after our trip to court a few years ago. She has subsequently changed her mind about this and a couple of days ago I received a letter from her outlining these changes. She writes that in the future she will want only one contact weekend each month. She elaborates no further and gives no reason for this sudden about turn. I might be tempted to make a guess about its possible cause but, of course, it would be nothing more than that: a guess.

A positive by-product of this development, if viewed as one parent's retreat or withdrawal, is that in some way I suppose it reinforces the bond between the remaining parent and child.

Once again it feels like a further confirmation, another small event in a series of small events in which we find our lives ever more firmly entwined. Father and daughter again, you and me, just like this. Is it relief or just a vague sense of gratification to occasionally experience in a life so full of doubt, reservation and scepticism, one solid, ineffable certainty?

There is of course a price to pay for this and without the respite of alternative weekends, the weeks do tend to drag sometimes and I find myself teetering on exhaustion occasionally. I'm prone to headaches and I lose the thread of sentences half-way through and forget simple everyday words. So I am particularly fortunate that, at this point in your life, you develop a completely new obsession. It seems to have come out of nowhere but for the last few months, you have become, like so many before you, absolutely fixated on Audrey Hepburn! Now, every evening after supper, nothing makes you happier than two hours or so spent in front of a DVD of *Roman Holiday*, *Funny Face*, *My Fair Lady* or any of the others. Films that you are quite content to watch over and over again.

This at least gives me a break every evening and I should say that I'm extremely grateful to Miss Hepburn for the wonderful opportunity she has provided me.

Actually I am of the opinion that there is something deeper going on here. I think on some level I am witnessing a process of assimilation and identification. I think to you she embodies your whole notion of 'lady', elegance, style, flair or whatever the word is and, beyond simply being a role model, I suppose she represents, in the mind of a young girl, a particular embodiment of the whole idea of femininity.

If your projection of yourself in Paris is of the artist, then your projection of yourself as a young woman is found in the films of Audrey Hepburn.

So the weekend arrives and I am due to ask my second question. I confess I am rather distracted first thing after breakfast when you inform me that you want a 'dress to sleep in'. This I find a particularly curious request until it is pointed out to me by someone in the know that this is Miss Hepburn's chosen night attire in *Roman Holiday*. I smile and tell you I'll keep a look out for you.

To be honest, I muse quietly as I make my way up the road to your godmother's house. I can't think of a single good reason why you shouldn't have a role model – even if you are actually asleep at the time.

Your godmother answers the door and I explain that I've come to ask her a question. Basically, I tell her that I have really come to offer her a job and she invites me in. My rehearsed preamble escapes me completely at this point and I just ask her if she would like to work with you for three days a week as your personal tutor. I explain that this would involve her working alongside your stepmother and that she would be mainly covering your academic needs and working long-term towards accreditation of some kind. I don't know if the money that we can offer her compares well with what she might expect working in a more orthodox environment but before I am even able to discuss terms she has already accepted. In fact, she seems altogether thrilled at the prospect.

She explains that for the past couple of years, being your teacher has always been her idea of the 'dream job'. Even based on those few sessions a couple of years ago, she really feels that with the right approach you are capable of doing some remarkable things, beyond even the achievements you have already made. Then she tells me that she is convinced that you should set your sights on GCSEs and nothing less. Even if it only means you get one or two, it would show, for all time and to all people, your level of intelligence.

This is the first time anyone has ever made a direct reference to anything specific of this nature to me and I actually find it rather frightening more than anything else.

While my mind is still processing all this information, she has another suggestion. As she is talking, I follow her into the small sunroom or conservatory that has been built on the rear of her house. Light and airy and not much bigger than a box room, it is currently strewn with cardboard boxes, crates and packing materials, lingering evidence of the recent move. She tells me she hadn't really decided what to do with the room as it was too small to be used as a secondary living room but it would make an absolutely perfect schoolroom for you.

She points and gestures and as she talks, I can see so clearly what she has in mind. The room is big enough for all your equipment and all the required resources, yet is small enough to create a good intimate working environment. It is a familiar place yet it is distinct from your home, and the schoolroom (and already I am referring to it as such) will be somewhere you come to work.

Your godmother seems delighted with this arrangement, perhaps it's the opportunity to put the room to some good use but I think if ever there was an ideal location for you to learn and flourish and be remarkable then this might very well be the place.

We arrange a date to begin a new term, which gives your godmother time to work out all her lesson plans and get the schoolroom ready. I return home and drag you away from *Breakfast at Tiffany's* to tell you the news.

My second question has two ticks and a star.

You are four years old and sadly we have to spend part of the day in your assessment centre. I remain on the premises, in fact I sit in the head teacher's office reading and making corrections to chapter 14 of my novel and occasionally answering the phone. Being in such an environment ensures that I'm constantly reminded of the fact that, in less than a year, you will be assessed and then go to the 'appropriate school' for your needs. There is a school in the borough that, as far as I understand, caters for children with primarily physical disabilities. Kids of reasonable intelligence with varying levels of other problems. That is the school I want for you and I have less than a year or so to make sure you get a place there.

Meanwhile, on a wet, overcast April morning, your assessment centre is darker and more foreboding than ever. I have grown to hate the all-pervading mood of resignation here. To me, there is a sense that everyone in the place – staff and children alike – have given up, abandoned everything aside from that brooding, resentful sense of futility. (Actually, I have always believed that it is this precise quality that is responsible for that miserable odour you so often encounter in public and civic buildings; down those waxed fluorescent corridors of the municipal dead.)

There is no heart here, no enthusiasm, no stimulation, too much blind acceptance and not enough possibility. That a child can be comprehensively assessed, or in truth can be *written off*, before the age of five might be viewed as progress but I am not convinced. These are probably the same values and attitudes that have been in place for a hundred years.

Everything seems to commence with that subtle erosion of dignity.

A day or so later I take you up to Guy's Hospital for an appointment with the orthopaedic surgeon and we listen to more bad news. You are to undergo major surgery on your hips.

'When?' I ask.

'Well,' he says, recoiling slightly – evidently this is the most ridiculous question he has ever heard. 'As soon as possible, I think, don't you?'

This doesn't exactly answer my question but I feel disinclined to push the matter.

We return home and in an attempt to lift our spirits we dance around the kitchen together to 'Sh-boom' by The Crew-Cuts.

Having subjected you to all manner of music in the past few years, I have noticed with some interest what does and what does not appeal to you. Generally speaking your tastes are eclectic and entirely unpredictable. I can never guess what will next spark your interest. There is no particular governing taste that I have so far witnessed. We used to listen to Mahler, Schubert and Shostakovich when I was writing articles. You

118

didn't seem to mind this in the least but *Il Travatore* used to drive you round the bend.

Recently, however, I have noticed that you have started to respond vocally to blues slide guitar. Last night I was listening to some pre-war compilation and while the music was playing – it was Bukka White or Son House I think – I could hear you making these little noises in time with the music. This is the only time I have ever heard you do this.

When you return to your day centre for your music therapy session, I chat to the therapist about this latest musical development. My own personal theory is that because the actual technique of playing with a bottleneck often produces half tones and even quarter tones, then musically it bears the greatest similarity to the cadences and patterns of human speech.

She smiles at my theory but looks unconvinced.

In the evening, perhaps worn out by your music therapy, you go to sleep quite early. On those rare occasions that I am able to watch you sleep I do sometimes experience an odd twinge of *something*. In your peaceful sleeping features there is no hint of the pain or of the drama that unfolds around you constantly. There is no hint of anything, just the calm beatitude of a sleeping little girl. There is no hint of anguish and what I am trying to clumsily avoid saying is that there is nothing obvious that suggests ... disability.

So I watch you dreaming your dreams, your private girl's dreams, and pray that whatever happens in them you might be treated with love and respect.

At this point in your life, the question I am asked with increasing regularity is 'are you going to have another child?' Some even add the somewhat over-familiar 'nice little brother or sister for Sophie'. I have come so close to overreacting to what I consider to be the vague implication of this question that I am only able to restrain myself with the greatest will-power.

A little *normal* baby, you mean! Another dull, ordinary child!

Some little scrap of safe, regular homogenised humanity unto whom I can hoist all my thwarted ambitions. Great idea! A drip-dry, boil-in-the-bag, modern, self-cleaning convenience infant. One who can be all those things that you will *never* be.

Invariably, I smile but say nothing.

Actually, I recall one of the very few things I have retained from doing Latin for two years: the expression '*De minimis non curat praetor*' (meaning something like 'Your petty laws don't apply to me').

You and I have an imaginary family crest that consists solely of those words.

The following week is another one of my tired weeks.

Scratchy.

Awkward.

Irritable.

Vile.

I walk through vague, dislocated days, the extremes of tiredness promoting a state of being not that far removed from drunkenness. I get these bouts periodically nowadays and I just feel so totally exhausted. A quite incredible tiredness, far beyond that which might be cured by A Good Night's Sleep. This is a deep, deep, sagging spiritual fatigue. You don't dream of a cure and you don't dream of recovery. You can only think about dragging yourself through the rest of the day.

During this particular week your music therapist rings me and we talk about the report she is writing about you. This report will be submitted to the Directorate of Education as part of the process leading up to the writing of your statement.

To give it its full title a Statement of Special Educational Needs is an official document that will set out a programme of education for the future. It takes into consideration all your problems and difficulties, yet will also hopefully help you to work towards your full potential. The former bit I imagine in your case will always be the far easier of the two.

All the teachers and therapists are requested to write reports

and I will actually be asked at some point to write one myself.
So much of your future hinges on this.

I am disappointed that the music therapist's report is cautious rather than glowing and I urge her to change it slightly. I know, and she does too, that a great deal now depends on her report. Without at least one really positive report, I fear I will again just be another deluded parent making claims on behalf of a child whose disabilities are too much for him to accept.

Meanwhile I am nearing the end of my novel. I still sit with you on my lap for an hour or so every day even when you have been at the assessment centre earlier. I do make a point of asking you every time if you want to come and help me and every day you use your 'yes' response. This way, at least, I don't feel that I'm forcing you to do something you find boring.

Strangely enough I ran into one of the old day centre staff last week and I was telling her about you sitting on my lap as I wrote. She told me a rather interesting story. They had a number of computers at the day centre and tried using one a couple of times with you without much success. They were trying to get you to use a switching system whereby you could build a picture of a house or a duck or something on the screen. You showed not the slightest interest in switches, screens or ducks and couldn't even be bothered to look at the monitor. Then, just as they were about to abandon the idea, the computer crashed and blocks of text were randomly shown on the screen.

Suddenly your eyes lit up and you were most interested, in fact you couldn't take your eyes off the screen. That's my girl!

You are four years and 51 days old and apart from your imminent hip operation this is the day I have been dreading. It is your first annual review and it takes place this afternoon at your assessment centre. Teachers and therapists, an educational psychologist who forms an essential if slightly vague part of the assessment process, and me sitting around talking about your future education.

This is the first time that I have had the chance to really talk about what I want for your future in practical educational terms. Obviously, so much is based upon how you are viewed now at the age of four, your achievements and more importantly your potential. You are non-mobile and non-verbal and judging your degree of understanding or your intelligence is always terribly difficult. In fact, this afternoon everybody seemed to preface every comment by remarking just how *difficult* it has all been.

With this degree of physical disability, a true assessment of a child is almost impossible and this afternoon I am offered informed speculation and inspired guesswork. I say that for the past year or so I have felt that the burden of proof has fallen to me to prove that you are a bright enough little girl. Given that most children with cerebral palsy have normal intelligence, shouldn't the burden have rested on those who doubt your intelligence?

The educational psychologist considers the question and then says slowly, 'You must realise that Sophie has extremely complex needs...'

Judging by the murmurs of approval, I seem to be the only person in the room who doesn't regard this as an answer.

Things progress downward from there. Despite a brave last-minute effort by the music therapist and her trusty video, the meeting ends without any conclusions being drawn. Nothing is finalised, more reports are needed. In essence, it is simple, I still need something, God only knows what, some hard, tangible evidence that will prove your level of understanding.

Just enough to give you a start.

Just enough to give you some degree of recognition.

If ultimately you fail the education system or it fails you, then at least I can feel that I honoured my side of the bargain. I didn't let you down. I did keep my promise.

Shortly after the review, I have an equally miserable case conference with your entire legal team in Lincoln's Inn Fields. In attendance at the conference with you, your mother and me are all the experts, solicitors and barristers. We all sit around a huge table and regard one another with quiet suspicion.

It is a depressing three hours. I disagree with a lot of what is said and everyone takes it in turns to disagree with me. All I learn is that the case will now take even longer than I thought.

At one point a junior barrister seems to take great delight in informing the assembly that it would be hard to judge what would have been your 'future earning potential' because 'the father hasn't had (chortle) what might be (chortle) termed a (chortle chortle) *normal career path*'.

When the general merriment subsides I inform one and all that I could make more money than everyone in the room put together by dealing in drugs and that therefore you shouldn't judge potential earnings simply on 'career paths'.

There follows a brief silence and I feel the point has been made. I just wish I hadn't been the one to make it.

I don't actually think it was a good idea for you to be present – you are talked about as if you were some hypothetical legal problem. You sit on my lap throughout but it is not long before I am having another one of my running away moments – this time, we sail our golden ship across distant azure seas, we discover new islands all of which will be named after you. I carry you along white sandy beaches, you are lighter than air, the essence of life itself. Great beautiful birds with brilliant plumage fly overhead calling out to us on the gentle breeze. As we bathe in rock pools, millions of tiny fish, darting, dazzling and brightly coloured, play and dance forever around our feet.

In such a fashion do I dream away three dreary hours.

The following weeks pass quickly and it is not long before we find ourselves on the 15th floor of Guy's Tower, one Sunday evening on the eve of a day when you will undergo major surgery on both hips. Your mother is working and so I have volunteered to stay with you during the weeks and she will take over at the weekends. Guy's Tower has breathtaking panoramic views across London and a man may contemplate many things. Except that on this particular evening this man would rather not.

We pass a predictably disturbed night and at about 8.15 the following morning I accompany you downstairs to the first floor, where the anaesthetist puts you under. I think you look worried so I hold your hand and talk to you.

'You must be brave.'

You blink.

'Actually, we both must be brave.'

You blink again.

The last thing I tell you before you surrender yourself to the anaesthetic is that I will always love you more than anything in the whole world.

If it is the last thing that you ever hear...

But I really must stop thinking like this.

You are wheeled away through double doors and I find myself alone back in the corridor. Everything suddenly seems absurd, nothing has any substance or the slightest relevance to me. Vague thoughts, doubts. The lifts to my right, the drink machine to my left, everything belongs to a different time and place. Statements, assessment centres, that other world, back *there*, back *then*, as remote suddenly as dinosaurs or Vikings.

You are actually having surgery to both hips, your dislocated right hip and your subluxed left. It is a fairly common condition in children with your problems, caused by the increased muscle tone and stiffness. The operation involves inserting a little 'metalwork' into the joint to prevent the hip dislocating again in the future. The operation will take about four and a half hours, but that is in their time. The expression 'four and a half' means as little to me as the expression 'hours'.

Eventually, word is sent back to the ward that you are in the recovery room and I chase back down to the first floor.

124

You are zonked out on painkillers but all is well apparently and I am told the operation all went according to plan. After a while, you slowly start to open your eyes. You look straight at me and start screaming at the top of your voice.

'That will be the pain,' a nurse helpfully explains. 'It's quite normal.'

I spend the following few nights in a cubicle. You are just around the corner in a cot on the main ward, where you remain after the operation so the nurses can keep an eye on you. (The staff here are very good; they tell me to go away and go back to sleep in the most polite way imaginable.) When the staff are confident they have your pain under control, you join me in the cubicle. You are being so brave and I am so proud of you. We have regular visits and check-ups and everyone is happy with your progress. But it's a slow process and time dawdles from hour to hour and from day to night.

Eventually, after a couple of weeks or so, your plaster cast is reinforced and finally we are driven home by ambulance. Lying in our hall is a letter from the Directorate of Education requesting from me a report on you. I throw myself into the task with improbable gusto. Finally, I think I will be part of this decision-making process. Yahoo! I have the chance to air my views, to make all the right points, to say what needs to be said, to stand up and make a difference. That is the fantasy – the reality is, I imagine, that the ramblings of a deluded parent are unlikely to be taken all that seriously.

The next few months drag rather slowly. It is basically a protracted period of convalescence, which lasts until your new spinal brace is fitted and collected. At this point we are able to discard the plaster cast and with it our memories of the summer.

One of the benefits of the surgery that is immediately apparent is that you are sleeping so much better now and you can tolerate a sitting position for far longer periods. I take you out for a spin in your new buggy every day and you seem to enjoy this enormously. I'm still doing the post-op exercises with you every morning and evening, but in the last weeks prior to your return to school, finding things to stimulate your interest for the rest of the day does sometimes become difficult. We have our buggy trips, I read to you, we look at art books, we listen to music and when you're in the mood we might do an hour or so on the computer. I think I am doing quite well under the circumstances but when your physiotherapist confirms that you are ready to return to your assessment centre, I catch myself breathing a secret sigh of relief.

You are four years and 194 days old and after a break of over four months, a combination of a summer holiday, the surgery to your hips and a lengthy convalescence, you finally return to your assessment centre. I admit I push you through the gates this morning with mixed feelings but everyone there seems incredibly pleased to see you again and one or two of the staff even smile at me.

In the lobby we are met by the headmistress who asks me into her office. With the least possible ceremony imaginable she blurts out that she has heard that the panel have made their decision and next year you will be going to the school that I so desperately wanted you to go to. This was the last thing I was expecting to hear and I am speechless.

I am everything-less.

I rush into the classroom where you are being read a less than riveting story about tooth decay or something and, apologising to staff and pupils alike, I take you out of your chair and dance up and down the corridor with you for five minutes.

This is a moment to cherish, I tell you, as we tango to a tune that plays only in my head, this is a moment I want us to remember for ever and ever. We did it! You showed them all how clever you are and now it's official.

The band put down their instruments, the tango grinds to a

halt and I return you to your classroom.

The future can wait.

All that matters is that I am not alone in believing in you and believing that one day you will prove yourself.

I am so proud of you.

I am proud of you every day.

But today is a special day for both of us.

The following week I am again chatting to the headmistress and she points out that when you start school full-time it will be good for me to have some free time again. This is a commonly held generalisation that I have heard from a number of people. Am I missing something here? Why will it be so much *better* for me when you are in school every day? They have no idea about you and me.

It was never just a one-way thing, you know.

You have taught me so much and saved me from ... well, me, I suppose. You have shown me to always look a little deeper, not to rely upon the obvious, the immediate or the visible. Even without traditional language, you and I have been communicating in our own way for almost five years.

You stopped me from falling head first into that netherworld, where everything has been vacuumed, disinfected, scrubbed and polished free of any meaning. A world where nothing has any essential quality or value and all the symbols and tokens, with which we surround ourselves, the very articles upon which we focus all desire, ultimately represent themselves and nothing else.

A valentine card means love.

So what then is love?

Love is simply that quality represented by a valentine card!

The mystery is drained away.

You have brought all the mystery back into my life and I am eternally grateful.

I don't view you going to school as an end to our time together. Our story doesn't end like that. Nothing ends like that, we are simply awaiting the next obstacle, the next challenge, it is not *over*, it will never be *over*.

Actually, it is impossible for there to be an *over*.

A month or so later, I take you in a cab to your new school, where you spend the morning in the reception class. You will be going in on Fridays and Tuesdays for the time being until you start full-time on your birthday next month.

I confess from the little that I have witnessed I am worried that your lessons (very academic, very national curriculum) might be just a little over your head at the moment. The contrast between the atmosphere in the classroom here and classrooms at your assessment centre could not be greater.

I worry that you might not be able to keep up.

Then a couple of evenings later I witness something so extraordinary that I can still hardly believe it myself.

I will draw no conclusions; I will restrict myself to facts.

I have spent most of the day taking my ailing computer to be fixed. Meanwhile, your mother decided that she'd like to see your school and so, having taken a day off work, she accompanies you to school and stays with you during your lesson. Today your class has been learning about the letter 'a'.

After your supper, as an experiment, to see how much of the lesson you have absorbed, your mother puts a pen in your hand and asks you if you can write down the letter you were shown earlier.

Your mother's method involves supporting your upper arm whilst leaving your hand free at all times. You commence by making a few scrawls on the paper, then a few more, then slowly the scrawls evolve and become more organised. I watch you moving your wrist very slightly as you gain more control.

After a dozen attempts one sees the start of a few primitive letter 'a's.

After a dozen further attempts I am presented with a piece of paper on which is written a definite legible letter 'a'.

I have stared at that piece of paper all evening.

It represents both an end and a beginning.

Over the following couple of weeks, your mother spends time with you every evening teaching you more letters. The process is agonisingly slow but you are developing your skill and technique every session. Meanwhile, I visit the school to chat to the head teacher about this development. For some reason, I thought this kind of ability would be quite common. (It makes a pleasing quasi-logical sense to me. The need to communicate being such a strong fundamental urge that, denied speech, it would find alternative methods.)

But I am wrong: it is not that common at all.

We discuss your background and home life and it is suggested that you sitting on my lap every day and watching me write might have had a significant role in developing your interest. This is obviously fairly unusual and certainly not a *normal* part of a *normal* child's *normal* day. The headmaster feels that this could be one of the key factors.

I tell him that fiction has so little purpose in most people's lives nowadays that it was nice to think that I was able to find a use for it, however unlikely.

You are five years old today and at 8.30 this morning I carry you on to the school bus and then watch from the window and wave as you are driven off. Not only do you start school full-time today, you also start travelling there on the school bus *on your own*. I watch the bus disappear from view as tears start running down my face. All parents go through this, I tell myself, and they probably do.

I look around the lounge, at the debris from where we unwrapped some of your presents this morning, and feel so overwhelmingly alone, so utterly useless. Then comes the panic. Help! I can no longer find any reason to justify my existence! I did once but you've gone to school now.

So, I take what I grandly consider to be a most positive step and post off two copies of the manuscript of my recently completed novel to a couple of publishers. I hand the two weighty packages across the counter at the post office and instantly regret it.

I am at your grandparents' house and not at home when you get back from school but your mother calls to tell me that you have had a good day in school, and before we all return for the birthday celebrations she wants to do some writing with you.

Then, just as we are preparing ourselves to leave, the phone rings again. It is your mother and she tells me that you have just written your first word.

The time is 5.28.

The word is 'big'.

And with that word a season passes as one will surely now begin.

You are thirteen years old and as the day falls on a Sunday we mark the occasion by hiring out a room in our local pub and inviting all our friends and family to join us for lunch. You sit at the centre of our group and the mood is informal and relaxed and you seem to enjoy yourself. You have some wonderful presents this year, virtually all of them relating to painting and art. Now that an emerging talent and passion has revealed itself again it is so much easier for people to choose a thoughtful and appropriate gift for you. I realise that for many years, this has often posed a slightly delicate problem.

I get into a number of discussions about your schooling and the new arrangement we are trying with your godmother in her schoolroom. Already the results have been pretty remarkable and I let your godmother tell a couple of stories about your mental maths skills that have so amazed and impressed her. She asserts that you are, in her opinion, definitely GCSE material. I shudder when she talks like this. I don't know why, I don't know if it's the level of expectation or the pressure it might put on you. Is it possible that on some level I am still seeking that all-important proof? Then once again I wonder who will benefit most from that proof. Is it still really that important? Either way, I am far happier when she goes on to recount the innumerable incidents when you have, despite urgent entreaties and encouragement, absolutely refused to use a calculator during maths lessons. The plan has always been for you to write instructions for its use, which is perfectly legitimate in an exam situation. But you are adamant about this and any discussion is pointless.

The general consensus is that you consider relying on a calculator to be cheating in some way. Furthermore, and to my mind possibly more signicantly, it denies you the great opportunity to show off your talents. We have all tried reasoning with you, explaining how much easier your lessons might be but you seem fairly intransigent on the subject. I suppose you want to do things on your own terms – just like you have always done.

It is rapidly becoming another one of those wonderful stories that have gathered around you over the years. Stories I will never weary of hearing or retelling.

Over the course of the day, it is pointed out to me fairly cheerlessly that you are now a teenager, as though this is something in itself to be feared. I'm sure there will be new challenges for me and you in the future just as I am certain there will be subtly modified or elaborately disguised versions of all the old ones.

But a season is surely passing again as I'm endlessly reminded that a new one is just beginning.

Fourth Season

Putting Dreams on Paper

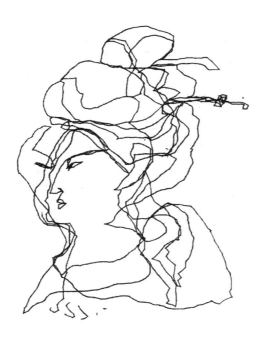

You are five years and 125 days old and we spend a warm August afternoon in the company of the woman who will subsequently be your personal teaching assistant and eventually your stepmother. Such identifiable roles are a little way off in the future and for the time being she is simply a family friend. Albeit, if this afternoon is any indication, one who seems to take enormous delight in taking you on swings, pushing you down slides and splashing around with you in paddling pools. She has a son your age and a slightly older daughter and she reasons, quite accurately as it happens, that you might have been denied such quintessential childhood experiences in the past. I confess that up until this moment, it is not something to which I ever gave a great deal of thought but I can certainly see how much you enjoy the time you spend in her company, and over the following weeks and months you develop a great rapport with one another.

We are coming to the end of your summer holiday, which although largely free of drama and incident has given your mother the chance to finish showing you the alphabet and various everyday words. For an hour or so every afternoon you now stand in your standing frame, a device that strengthens the muscles in your legs and increases your weight-bearing ability. It's an ungainly and rather ugly piece of equipment but it does the job. It arrived at the start of the summer and took up residency in our lounge. However, I must say you do seem to enjoy being vertical and as it means that both your arms are free it also puts you in the ideal position to write. Your mother has taken full advantage of this posture and, while you are standing, she puts a pen in your hand, supports your upper arm and holds the paper for you to write.

Your progress has been impressive and you are now writing in short abbreviated, idiosyncratic sentences exclusively in lower case. There is obviously a considerable amount of effort involved and at the moment you can usually only manage an hour each day before you are exhausted. But it's gratifying beyond words to see you write something as simple as 'want food'.

We are hoping that at the start of term we will be able to show one of the classroom assistants how to write with you when you are in school. This would allow you to take a much more active part in your lessons.

With a certain pride, I note that you are now regularly referring to 'mummi' and 'daddi'. This quirk of spelling that will continue, results from your mother's haste to include us in your vocabulary prior to getting as far as 'Y' in her progress through the alphabet. But it's heartening to be referred to in the conversation, particularly when one afternoon, I am presented with a piece of paper on which are written the words 'daddi love me'.

At the moment I just observe the process, partly because, having finally succumbed to the frequently voiced conventional wisdom, I realise that it's beneficial for you to spend some time with your mother and for the two of you to work together on something like this. But it is strenuous work for the pair of you and having a splash in a paddling pool every so often is certainly no more than you deserve.

Your grandma is also now starting to take advantage of your developing abilities. She too has started writing with you and it's interesting to note that you form your letters in precisely the same way as you do with your mother and you maintain your unique shorthand syntax in an identical manner. But as well as this, your grandma has started trying to draw with you. At this stage it is just another way of playing with a pen but it's something you are enjoying enormously.

Meanwhile 'daddi', whilst not actively involved with your writing at this stage, finds himself with time on his hands, enjoying a few weeks' respite. Except that I find it hard to just switch off and relax. In my quieter moments away from you, I seem only able to reflect upon our current situation and make some sort of provision for the next challenge we might face. This life can be exhausting, shattering, saddening, heartbreaking, upsetting and infuriating; it can drive a person to the very limits of patience and endurance and even sanity but when I am given a break from it, I find it hard to walk away from you or take any advantage of the opportunity offered me.

Around this time, I manage to find a publisher for my novel, something I am absolutely thrilled about but still I feel that writing is just something that I do in the gaps in our life together. Furthermore, there is nothing I will ever write that could rival for significance and purity that which you are now writing with your mother every afternoon.

When you finally return to school it is only a matter of hours before the latest challenge is unveiled to me. This challenge comes in the form of a word. The word is VALIDATION and it is handed to me with little ceremony one afternoon when I am called in to see your new class teacher. Over the months and years I will learn to hate and despise this word; it will track me and stalk me and darken so many days but this afternoon I simply enquire what exactly it is that requires validation.

Sometimes I am so incensed or I become defiant and angry, sometimes I want to scream and shout out against ignorance and stupidity. But there are the other times, like this afternoon, when I just feel another weary line etch itself across my face, while somewhere in some cold, dark sound-proofed compartment of the brain or the soul or whatever it is, there comes a great long lingering scream that no one will ever hear.

I listen politely as I am told that your writing will need validation before it is actually accepted as being your work and your work alone. Apparently there have been reported cases when children have written 'with help' (the term I learn today is 'facilitated writing'), when the helper has actually been moving the child's hand. This strikes me as a particularly evil thing to do; a child has the chance to communicate and it's abused in this fashion. I enquire why anyone would do this to a child and am told that sometimes people have problems dealing with their children's disabilities.

Another silent scream.

Another deep furrow.

Anyway, before your writing is accepted as being genuine it will need to be validated. This I learn can be achieved formally or informally. The formal version is a single test whereas an informal validation takes place over a period of months. The school, it seems, are keen to try the second alternative. There are many criteria for validation; one of the most common would be you passing on information to your helper that is accurate and correct and yet entirely unknown to the helper. An example of this was when you wrote 'must feed dog' with your mother at the end of last term. She queried this the following day with your class teacher who explained that she had told the class that she was going on holiday and that she wasn't taking her dog with her. She had neglected to mention the dog was actually staying at a kennel. You had, in that instance, been passing on information unknown to your mother and so that would qualify as an example of an informal validation.

It is suggested that we have a meeting later in the week during which they will very closely observe you writing.

In short, I think I am being told that they don't believe us. That they think your mother is moving your arm for you and making you write. They dress this accusation in words like 'exercising undue influence' but it amounts to much the same thing. Once again I am faced with the daunting task of presenting proof. I thought we had finally stumbled upon our miracle – the method that would prove your intelligence beyond any question once and for all. Now it seems I am being called upon to prove the veracity of the actual method itself.

The miracle is thus tarnished, is judged illusory.

Beyond this, and perhaps this is even harder to endure, it has placed a real doubt in my mind. I am not entirely relishing the experience but I can see how the school might have come to their conclusions, how it may appear to an outsider. Given the background, I suppose it might all seem a little dubious. I suppose I was naïve to think that anyone would just take our word for it. Not when there is such a given about the parents of disabled children.

In the evening, after she returns from work, your mother has another writing session with you and at its conclusion I am informed that you 'want buy daddi dog'. I smile and I thank you for your kind thought but at the moment there is such a great shadow being cast over all this I find myself close to tears. It's another one of those times when I don't know what to feel, what to think or what to say.

That same old numbness.

After you've gone to bed, I talk to your mother and explain the situation to her and how your writing requires validation. She is frankly horrified by the suggestion and dismisses the very idea that she might be helping you. I explain that the school has arranged an appointment for us so they can scrutinise the method involved in the writing and your mother simply shrugs. It is as though the whole matter is of no consequence to her and should be of no more consequence to me.

After six years of marriage, of all the things I envy about your mother, I think uppermost is her utter certainty. Most often manifested as a sort of strict pragmatism, there are moments, like this evening, when some comfort might be drawn from it.

I had been telling you that I was going to start writing with you soon, just a little chat now and again. Nothing significant, just a friendly hello every so often but I don't even feel like doing that at the moment. If there's any chance that I might move your hand or make you write something that you don't want to I would never forgive myself. I find it sad that I'm denying myself a great opportunity but the thought of even accidentally helping you is a horrible thing to contemplate.

By the time I make my way to the meeting, after mulling it over for a day or two, I have decided that there are three possible outcomes. That you are actually writing. That your mother is helping you write. Or that some of it is you and some of it is your mother – the proportions of which are undetermined but sufficient to undermine the entire process.

The odds, as ever, seem weighed heavily against you.

The meeting takes place in your classroom after school and is attended by you, your mother and me, your class teacher and your new speech therapist, to whom I am introduced at the start of the meeting. After the briefest of formalities, you are placed in the standing frame and with your mother's help you begin to write. You inform us that you are tired and you want to go home. This strikes me as an extremely good idea but they are not finished with you yet. They want to try a quick validation test. The speech therapist and I observe as your mother is asked to leave the room while your class teacher tells you a word. Your mother is then asked to return and you are requested to write down the word you have just been told.

The word was 'cup'.

But you do not write this.

Instead, you write, 'you mad.'

To be fair, this neither proves nor disproves your ability or our claims on your behalf but the school has seen enough. They have been presented with no real evidence at this stage to reinforce the idea that you are writing independently. However, they assure us that they will attempt to write with you in the demonstrated method. Although they then spend the remainder of the meeting suggesting that some method is found to enable you to communicate using switches and a computer.

As we are preparing to leave, the speech therapist tells me that she sympathises and understands, that she realises how much as parents we would like you to be able to write. 'It's a perfectly natural response,' she offers by way of reassurance.

I smile but somehow I don't seem able to find the right words to express exactly how I feel at this moment.

You are five years and 224 days old and as we approach the Christmas holidays, I receive a phone call from your speech therapist. She asks if I can call in and see her at the school later in the week. There is something she wishes to discuss with me 'face to face' as she puts it.

I confess that I'm quite baffled as to what might lie behind this request. I don't think that I have had any contact with her since that fateful meeting back in September. In fact, there has been very little contact of note with the school either. You are continuing to regularly write with your mother and your grandma and any evidence of 'informal validation' I am careful to make note of.

Beyond that, I am also very mindful of you writing things that might be inappropriate or too far beyond your experience and, in doing so, I realise how much I have started to view your progress objectively. From *their* point of view. This is something I have noticed happening in myself in recent weeks – prompted initially I imagine by that same meeting. I catch myself observing you and our situation from an outsider's perspective. No longer am I relying on pure faith as I realise that faith will only take you so far. It saddens me greatly and I feel most acutely that I am letting you down in some way but I have started to see things in terms of tangible proof and concrete evidence.

Something I can hold in my hand.

To throw straight back in the face of anyone who ever doubts you in the future!

Over the past few weeks or so I have also, very cautiously, started to write with you. I admit I found it terribly difficult at first. I was so worried that I might influence what you were writing that I supported your arm in such a forceful manner that it was absolutely impossible for you to move. Later, I learned to relax a little and we are now having the occasional chat. In the main I restrict myself to yes/no questions and very rarely anything beyond that. I might ask you to choose what you might like for supper but that's as deep as it gets at the moment.

I arrive at the school for my meeting and am shown into a small office. I briefly take in and mentally digest the unfamiliar surroundings, before I am joined by the speech and language therapist. She offers me a coffee, which I decline, and she seems hesitant, worried even.

She asks if you are looking forward to Christmas and we chat for a minute or two. I am very careful not to say anything contentious or inflammatory and just as I am about to enquire why she asked to see me, she asks me a question.

She looks at me intently and enquires in a nervous flurry if you always have a pen and paper with you when you are taken out.

I tell her that if we are going to be out for longer than a matter of a few minutes, then I would usually take a pen and paper for you.

'Good ... good,' she says with a smile that seems to express quite genuine relief.

Incredibly, she then goes on to explain that she was writing with you earlier in the week and you wrote that you felt 'frustrated' if you were out somewhere and didn't have the means to write with you. Before I can even begin to process this relatively simple piece of information, she is quickly apologising for being less than positive about your abilities back in September. She explains that she'd had a few attempts with little or no success and then suddenly the words became more recognisable. Ever since then she's been writing with you every chance she has.

I just about manage to stop myself trying to kiss her!

But she is not finished. She also points out that, for a five-year-old, 'frustrated' is a very advanced emotion. To show an understanding of the idea and use it in context would be impressive in any able-bodied child. At this point she proudly hands over the piece of paper and I can see the word in your instantly recognisable script.

She explains that she worries that you will not reach your true potential in the classroom unless someone is on hand to write with you all the time. Some of the classroom assistants have a go from time to time but it's not at anything like a consistent level. She suggests I get on to the Directorate of Education and request that they provide you with someone who can write with you all the time. In the meantime, I suggest that when we have meetings to discuss your progress, we are allowed to include examples of the work you do at home. She thinks this would be the fairest way to proceed.

She seems keen, desperate even, to distance herself from her own opinions of a few months ago and it is hard not to admire her for this. I hesitate to use the word 'conversion' (I do alarm myself periodically by how often, when talking about you, I lapse into the hyperbole and rhetoric of orthodox religion) but I sense that this is something that she feels very strongly about.

She continues to talk and sounds genuinely excited about the prospect of working with you in the future and talks about different ways of using your ability. At one points she suggests quite seriously that you may like to try your hand at writing poetry. She points out how well you express yourself and how concisely you write. Poetry might be a further creative means of expression for you, particularly as you may be able to put your ideas across in a matter of a few lines. This is an important consideration as the physical act of writing, as has already been discovered, is long-winded, laborious and exhausting for you.

The meeting comes to its natural conclusion at this point and I thank her for taking the time to talk to me and for all the work that she has been doing with you. She sounds a note of caution and once again, citing herself as an example, she reminds me that there will always be people who will doubt you and mistrust some of the claims made on your behalf.

Not *proof* exactly, I think as I make my way to collect you from your classroom and take you home. But beyond all doubt, I am certain that I have just been present at a fairly significant event.

You are thirteen years and 123 days old and for the very first time you draw a picture with your godmother, who will henceforth in our story be referred to as your tutor – as my failure to do this might be regarded as some kind of professional slight. The picture you have produced is a line drawing of a vase of flowers and a fine example of your usual style. But beyond this, it is also the first time that you have ever drawn with anyone other than your grandma.

You both seem particularly pleased with this development as it immediately adds a possible further dimension to your school day. Maybe in future, an hour's drawing will serve as a simple incentive or a reward at the end of a day's hard work. Naturally, as my mind is trained in its own particular way, I can't help but view the episode as a further validation. I notice instantly that your own very individual technique seems remarkably consistent regardless of who is assisting, and, by her own admission, your tutor, whilst having a great love of art, has absolutely no talents in that direction herself.

This is, I am confident, all your own work.

Over the next couple of weeks you continue drawing and produce a series of flower pictures, a subject for which you have always shown a particular flair. They seem like finished works and you are happy to leave them as they are rather than paint over them. Working with your tutor, you quickly devise a system and a technique to ensure that you have complete and total control over your own work. For example, when you are satisfied that your drawing is complete, you will simply stop at the end of a line and sign your initials.

Picasso once famously explored the possibility of drawing a picture without removing his pen from the paper so that the finished work is one continuous line. You have a book about these images, which we've often looked at, and this seems to have been a great influence. It is fairly easy to see that your drawing technique is your own version of this method. It is a skill that you continue to develop and the amount of planning involved as you approach a blank page remains a quite remarkable talent in itself.

Even by the standards you have set yourself, your work seems to have shifted a gear or two of late and I think it's fair to say that the degree of empathy involved in a creative working relationship of this kind will only enhance the bond between pupil and teacher.

Meanwhile, on most days you can be found at the schoolroom with your stepmother and your tutor working your way through a fairly vigorous schedule. You are still point-blank refusing to use a calculator but, in your defence, it should be pointed out that you do seem to be doing fairly well without one. Your mental maths skills are as impressive as ever and I imagine these are some of the resources you depend upon whenever you are planning to draw and to cover an entire surface with a single line.

This first term you are also studying Ghandi and Ché Guevara and the resulting debates I am told have been 'lively'.

As your days at the schoolroom have given me back a couple of hours, I often take myself off on my bike for an hour or so. Sometimes I may have some underlying reason or vague purpose for cycling somewhere but this is rare. More often than not I just pedal around the place aimlessly enjoying the peace and the countryside.

One day, a few weeks into the new term, I am cycling through a nearby village and something pinned to a notice board outside the post office catches my eye. I get off my bike and hurry over to read it. The small poster is announcing an annual art exhibition at the village hall in a few weeks. It invites submissions from local artists, local in this case being defined as no more than five miles away and luckily we just about qualify. The poster goes on to state that the organisers particularly welcome submissions from children and young people. I take a sudden lungful of air through my gaping mouth as I read the words over again as though half expecting that on subsequent readings they will rearrange themselves into a more mundane order. But submissions from children and young people are definitely welcome. There is a phone number and a website both of which I scribble down frantically before cycling home at a noticeably increased velocity.

After school, having visited the website and printed out an entry form, I put the idea to you. I suggest that you submit some of your recent pictures (the permitted maximum is three works) and hopefully they will find some space to exhibit them. This suddenly sounds like a very bold step and once again I worry that I might be putting pressure on you or that I'm simply setting you up to be disappointed. Painting is a marvellous and worthy outlet but thus far it has been an essentially private one. This would put it on a much more public stage. Besides, I would hate your pictures to be judged on anything other than their artistic merit and I will not have your work regarded as a titillating novelty in some way because the artist is so severely disabled. You, however, seem absolutely delighted by the prospect. We chat about it for a while and I realise how important this is for you.

It is a chance for you to declare yourself an artist in your own eyes.

Naturally, I am tempted to sound a note of caution, to remind you that we are only submitting pictures and that there is no guarantee that they will even be exhibited. But I stop myself, swayed mainly by your evident excitement and by my fear of once again reworking for the millionth time Max Miller's plough joke. Instead, I tell you that we should go through your pictures and select the best examples.

Over the next few days when you're not at the schoolroom, we work our way through your portfolio – I confess that I have never used this term before but, if you're going to be an artist submitting your work to exhibitions, I tell you that this might be a good time to start. Taken *en masse* in this manner you have built up such an impressive oeuvre (see portfolio) and there are so many single examples that I think are worthy of being exhibited.

Eventually, the selections are made by a committee consisting of the two of us in conjunction with your stepmother, your tutor and your grandma. After some deliberation, it is decided that you should submit two flower pictures and a landscape and eventually some sort of agreement is reached. When the pictures are framed, I complete the entry form and print a couple of labels to stick on the rear of the frames. Following the conditions of entry, these should show the title of the work, which is simple enough, together with the price, which is rather more complicated. I presume this is just a formality and explain that it might be better just to write 'not for sale', but you have very different ideas.

I point out that as it is a small local exhibition there are unlikely to be many sales and besides, I imagined that you might want to hang on to your paintings. In this, it seems, I am completely mistaken. You are quite happy to offer all the pictures for sale and have no particular attachment to any of your paintings. Once a picture is completed, you are finished with it and you simply move on to the next one. I don't know if this rejection stems from a sort of perfectionism but you will remain fairly consistent in this.

So, feeling your keen gaze upon me, I write what I consider to be a fairly reasonable price, neither modest nor extravagant, on the rear of all three paintings.

147

You are thirteen years and 175 days old and I am a witness to what I believe will prove to be one of the defining moments in your life.

A couple of days prior to this noteworthy event, on the allocated day for submissions, we take your paintings down to the village hall and pass them over to the organisers. It is a fair-sized hall and its white interior walls lend it a suitable ambience for an exhibition of this kind. Your details are noted and you are thanked for submitting your work. As we leave, we are assured that they will try and hang your pictures but, at this stage, they cannot guarantee anything more than that.

The following days pass quickly and on the day that we plan to visit the exhibition you are agitated and excited from the minute you wake up. All morning you are restless and distracted and seem to find it difficult to concentrate on anything, even giving you a drink is a struggle. There is little or no doubt what lies behind this sudden mood of infectious exuberance, and despite my usual tendencies, I find that I am disinclined to start lecturing you too heartily on the virtues of caution. But even writing with you proves problematic today and it is hard to actually decipher what you are trying to say, beyond the fact that I can distinctly make out the words 'an artist' at one point.

So following an utterly hopeless attempt to feed you lunch, we make our way to the exhibition. I make the fairly obvious sartorial decision of putting you in your beret for the occasion. We are accompanied by your stepmother and your tutor and, as we arrive at the hall, I whisper to your stepmother to sneak in quickly and make sure that your paintings are on display while I put you in your wheelchair. She returns a moment later and confirms with an expression of some relief that all three are on view.

Then she enquires about the little orange stickers. There are only a few dotted around the exhibition but all your pictures have them. I shrug but I do not dare to answer her question;

I know what those stickers usually mean but perhaps, I tell myself, it is different in a little local exhibition like this. But for the following 30 seconds I force my mind to remain blank as I push you into the exhibition.

Immediately, the organiser greets our arrival with a hearty 'congratulations' and this provides me with all the confirmation I need. In the most measured tones possible under the circumstances, I tell you that you have sold all three of your pictures! There have been a few sales here and there at the exhibition but you are the only artist to sell all three of his or her works.

Some of the people involved with the show come up to you and congratulate you and reiterate that it is an amazing accomplishment in an artist so young. Your pictures were displayed with several hundred other works and yet no one came close to matching your achievement. In fact, we are handed a piece of paper with the names and phone numbers of people who were too late to buy one of your flower pictures but would like to commission you to paint another one.

Today, I do not take my usual place alongside you, not now, not at this time. For this is your moment and I must line myself up with those ranks of people who regard you this afternoon with a combination of esteem and wonder. Not only did you announce to yourself that you were an artist, you have just proclaimed the fact to the entire world.

That's my daughter. She is an artist.

Tears come quickly this afternoon. Especially when I take your photo in front of your pictures. Your expression is wonderful, a curious combination of beatific joy and the slightest suggestion of a smug 'I told you so'.

And of course you did. Didn't you?

As we are leaving, one of the organisers informs me that the local press are showing a great interest in your success. He asks if he might pass on our details. I give him the required information and the following day we are visited at home by

149

a reporter and a photographer. We chat for an hour or so and I stress the significance of the exhibition; that your paintings were sold entirely on their own merit, that it was your talents and abilities that placed you on an equal footing with all the other artists in the area and that, for one day at least, your disabilities were of secondary importance. I also make the point that this success has confirmed your belief in yourself as an artist and the importance of this cannot be over-stressed.

Although you are no stranger to the press, this particular piece will be different. It will celebrate your talents and your skills and not simply your bravery or your endurance.

You are quite delighted with all the attention and you deserve every second of it. The article will consolidate your triumph and will remain forever embedded in this quite extraordinary sequence of moments. The piece will run the following week alongside a full colour photo of you looking at a recent painting of red roses. The general tone of the article will be glowing and the bold caption above it will read:

TALENTED SOPHIE
OUTSELLS THE REST
AT FESTIVAL SHOW

You are six years old and we arrange a small party at our house to celebrate your birthday. A couple of dozen friends and family join us for the afternoon and we all have a grand birthday tea in your honour. You have been a little under the weather recently but you perk up for the occasion and you seem to enjoy yourself. This is your first birthday since you have been able to communicate and I notice that so many of your presents this year reflect this change in our awareness. This increase in understanding has allowed you to develop and grow up in our eyes and I am delighted that so many of the books and tapes you are given today reflect something in which you have already expressed an interest, or actually indicated a desire to own.

I don't know if attaining six years qualifies as a notable stage in your development but your most frequently voiced complaint nowadays is that a certain item or activity is 'too baby' for you.

I want to mark your birthday this year for a number of reasons, but particularly because its significance might well be overshadowed by another date, about six weeks in the future; the day when the claim against the Health Authority is scheduled to be heard at the High Court.

For the past few weeks there has been a notable increase in activity. Aside from a number of meetings with your solicitor, I have also had discussions with barristers and accountants and they have all been having meetings with each other.

It is all getting rather intense and at this precise moment the overall effect is that your life seems to be taking place at some distance away from you.

We have been visited at home by a whole series of expert witnesses, some of whom are visiting for a second or even third time. I refrain from making my usual great claims on your behalf, from recounting oft-told anecdotes that serve to illustrate your intelligence. In a strange way, I actually feel disloyal but they are, as I am not infrequently reminded, the experts. Also, as I have been instructed, I make every effort to be helpful and co-operative with our visitors but I must confess that it does become a little wearisome after a while. But there are occasionally moments of respite from the general tedium.

One such moment occurred a few days ago during the visit of one of the Health Authority's experts. She asks me at one point if you ever demonstrate what she terms 'purposeful hand movements'. Naturally, I reply somewhat awkwardly that you can write and promptly wince as I anticipate a certain professional incredulity. I am therefore delighted when she explains that such a development doesn't surprise her in the slightest and that she has recently seen a young girl with a very similar range of difficulties who was writing in exactly the same way. Like you, this young girl is ambidextrous. In fact, she says, she was

151

going to ask me if we had attempted writing with you. This little piece of information from such an unlikely source cheers me up enormously for some reason.

While we're on the subject, I should mention that your solicitor has made the point on several occasions that your ability to write will have very little effect on the outcome of the case or your claim as, in the long-term, such an ability does not equate to any reduction in the need for future care.

Meanwhile, there has been no progress whatsoever in my attempt to get your school to provide you with someone to help you to write during lessons. Although I have discovered that the actual term for such a person would be a 1:1 Support Assistant. In my silly utopian naïvety, I once believed that in special needs education, once a need was identified, the help was provided. Sadly I now realise that such thinking is laughably child-like. It is nowhere near as simple as that and it takes a very long time for the process to reach a conclusion. Sadly, you have changed classes recently and your current class teacher, having failed to produce anything legible in her attempts to write with you, has declared herself thoroughly unconvinced by the claims made on your behalf. She is just the latest in a long line of doubtless well-meaning professionals who will adopt this stance with you. It is a line that stretches back almost to your very birth.

Of course, your speech therapist remains convinced of your abilities and I get regular reports from her of the limited contact she has with you. But while a doubt remains, the official line is that the Directorate of Education cannot commit itself to funding any extra staff 'at this time'. Naturally, I have arranged a couple of meetings and I've written a few letters but realistically I know that I have very little chance of shifting opinion on my own.

However, there has been one recent development regarding your education that I confess I could not have anticipated. It is not a daily or even weekly occurrence but fairly regularly, a couple of times a month on average, I will get a call from the school nurse informing me that you are in the medical room and that you are unwell. Naturally, the first time this happens I rush to the school and collect you and bring you home. As soon as we are back in the house, I am delighted, but a little surprised, to see you smiling and looking absolutely content. I put you in your standing frame, put a pen in your hand and ask you what the matter was, was it your back, did you feel sick, was there a pain somewhere, are you feeling tired, were you hot?

You smile and think for a moment and then write a single word: 'bored'.

All the subsequent incidents invariably follow this same pattern; I will get the call from the nurse, although I'm sure I can detect a certain ironic tone in her voice when she informs me that you are 'unwell again'. I will make my way to the school and collect you from the medical room and by the time you are home again you are perfectly happy once more. I will ask what the matter is if only for the chance to give you voice to your grievances.

'bored.'

I know I shouldn't actively approve of your moral descent into truancy or encourage this sort of behaviour but it's hard not to admire you for taking such direct action. With even the most limited physical abilities, you found a way to make your point; you registered a complaint, you protested. I don't think anyone aware of your particular situation in school at the moment could possibly be anything less than entirely sympathetic to your cause. It has certainly brought to my attention the extent of the problem. I don't blame you at all; I imagine you are incredibly bored.

It is around this time that I am handed the additional diversion of my first novel being published. As a way of expressing my belated gratitude, I dedicate every penny of my royalties to your old music therapy department. (In time, the book will make enough money for the department to renew their video equipment.) The book gets a couple of reviews and there are one or two features in the local press covering the music therapy story. One of these is accompanied by a photograph of you with your music therapist; it is the first time you have got your picture in the paper. It will not be the last.

I think you look particularly beautiful.

I do a few radio interviews to promote the book; most take place in London but I do find myself in Cardiff at one point doing a radio show at nine in the morning. The interviewer asks me about you and the music therapy angle and, for the first time in my life, I find myself talking publicly about us and our lives together. It is evidently a far more interesting topic than my novel as the succeeding line of questioning centres entirely on you.

As I talk about you two things occur to me. Firstly, I don't actually enjoy doing this sort of thing very much at all and secondly, I want to come home and tell you all about it.

I'm bored and I think that you of all people might be sympathetic.

You are six years and 61 days old when I receive a phone call around lunchtime from your solicitor. As was correctly predicted a week or so ago, the Health Authority has just made us an offer to settle your case. It is explained to me that this is common practice with our scheduled day in court less than a week away. Your solicitor is evidently far more experienced in these situations and when I am told that we will be declining this first offer, I am happy to leave the matter in more experienced hands. I am told that, without the slightest doubt, they will improve their offer and I will get another phone call when they do.

Sure enough, an hour or so later I receive a call and am informed that here has been another offer. Again the offer will be rejected. Apparently, there is always a degree of brinkmanship when a case reaches this point; indeed I recall being warned about it at our last meeting. The idea is to settle for the best possible offer calculated roughly on recent similar cases.

There are further phone calls and further updates and it is not long before I abandon myself to an afternoon of nail biting and pacing, terrified to stray too far away from the phone. I have been so involved with virtually every aspect of your life for almost every day of your six years but this afternoon is one of those times, surgery was another obvious instance, when I am reduced to the role of an agitated spectator. It is not a pleasant sensation in the slightest. At about half past three, I rush out and collect you from the school bus and rush back into the house again. I explain to you while we have our chat what is happening this afternoon and why your father appears to be afflicted with some nameless nervous mania.

Finally, as I am feeding you your supper, I answer the phone and I am informed that the case has been settled. (I should perhaps throw in a couple of exclamation marks at this point but it's been a long afternoon and I'm exhausted.) Your solicitor tells me that the Health Authority's last offer has now been accepted. Everyone is delighted with the outcome and, although I'm relieved that the case is settled, I can't really focus my mind on the full implications of what has just happened. The most appealing aspect of all this, I confess, is that we are not going to have to go to court next week after all.

In this, it seems I couldn't be more wrong.

It is something of a formality but on the allotted date we are still requested to attend court, where I presume the terms of the settlement are made legal and official.

So, the following Monday morning, after seeing you on to the school bus, your mother and I make our way into town to the Royal Courts of Justice on the Strand. We speak very little during the trip but I sense that we both share a similar apprehension and a strong will for the whole morning to be behind us. We are actually in court for a little over an hour, which is largely taken up with legal procedures. At one point, the barristers from both sides make fairly brief concluding speeches and I am stunned when, the barrister acting on behalf of the Health Authority, actually apologises to us for the mistakes made during your delivery. By glancing quickly to my right at your solicitor's face, I gather that this is by no means a common occurrence.

Whether it is this apology, the solemnity of the occasion, or the realisation that today marks the end of six long years, during which I had to continually remind myself that it was all for your benefit, I feel a tear come to my eye. Then, as the judge speaks prior to approving the settlement, he compliments your mother and I for all the work we have done and briefly singles out my particular contribution as being your main carer. His voice is reassuring and wise and comforting and kind and now the tears start rolling down my cheeks.

Twenty minutes or so later I have composed myself; we are back outside on the Strand and it is all over. Your mother returns home while I go for a coffee with our whole legal team. We discuss the timetable for the next few months and your immediate financial needs. Then, as I am heading back towards the station, your solicitor warns me that either later today or tomorrow I will probably be visited by the press. I am advised that it is better to be co-operative and talk to them.

I am back at home for barely an hour before I have to answer the door to a couple of reporters from a national newspaper. They want to talk about the case and so I invite them in. I am doing my best to be polite but it's not easy, as I have always hated the way these cases are usually reported in the press. The interview progresses along predictable lines and, judging by their very rigid line of questioning, I get the impression that they would far rather be talking to the money than wasting their time listening to what I have to say.

But, all things considered, I think I am doing reasonably well until one of them asks me to clarify the precise sum of the 'compensation'. I explain that the term is actually misleading in this case; this is not simply a lump sum of money paid to someone for an injury, the money that was awarded today is held in trust and will be used to finance extra help and equipment as it is needed in the future.

The interview sort of grinds to a halt at this point and instead of waiting until you come back from school, they suddenly remember a prior engagement and say their farewells. I study the press for the next couple of days and am not in the least surprised to find not a single mention of you or the case. Or indeed the 'compensation'.

The story is, however, picked up by the local press and the following week you actually make the front page of one paper. The headline reads:

CASH AWARD
FOR
BRAVE GIRL

I read all the articles out to you and you seem delighted to be once again the centre of attention. I tell you that you are a brave girl and that look here, it's not just me who thinks so.

Now everyone will know.

Over the next few months we get an indication of what a difference the money will make to your future. There are the more obvious aspects like searching around for a bigger house. Lacking any particular urgency, we've been doing this rather casually for a while now. We are looking for somewhere with an extra room or two on the ground floor that can be converted into a bedroom for you. As I am scanning the latest batch of estate agents' particulars, I realise that at some point in the past couple of years I have accepted the fact that you will never walk or be capable of dressing or looking after your self. As I don't recall a sudden dramatic realisation or one great heartbreaking moment when this occurred to me, I presume that such an awakening, like so many other aspects to being your father, is simply a slow process of reluctant and gradual assimilation.

But having accepted it, I find in myself, quite unexpectedly, a sense of steely pragmatism and it simply becomes a question of practicalities.

I also try again with your school and raise the question of getting you a personal support assistant to help you write and to generally contribute to lessons. Again, I explain to your head teacher that without such help, you are simply an observer. The response is not wholly unanticipated; because of the lingering controversy about the writing, while it lacks validation, the school does not think that the resources would be made available.

So we go into Plan B.

The one I've been mulling over for a few weeks.

A deep breath and I launch right into it.

I ask if the school would have any objections in principle if we funded a personal assistant ourselves? A person in that role would enable you to write all the time, to be available when you have something to say and cover all your personal care needs while you were in school. That way you would be far better equipped to join in with class activities and take an active part in lessons.

I prepare myself for the usual obfuscations and objections followed by the usual very kindly, very understanding flat out refusal. So, I confess I am somewhat stunned on this occasion when the head teacher informs me that such a thing is not at all uncommon. In fact, he tells me that there have been a couple of pupils in the school in the past who have had a privately funded assistant. I wince at the term 'privately funded' but realise that I am going to have to overcome these deep-rooted issues of personal principle and politics if I am going to claim, with any honesty, that I am acting solely in your best interests.

I return home and call your solicitor. I enquire if I would be able to employ (and I'm not sure I like that word either) an assistant to work with you in school. They would have no problem with this but enquire if I have anyone in mind and truthfully I say that I know someone who would be just perfect for the job.

So, a couple of months later at the start of the autumn term you return to school, driven by your new assistant: your special friend who pushes you down slides and plays in paddling pools with you. It marks the very beginning of an incredible partnership, one that will see you make extraordinary progress and take you so far beyond anyone's previous expectations. Your assistant has always been very supportive and very vocal in her belief in you and if anyone was an ideal candidate then surely it was her. Your paths first crossed several years ago when your grandma and grandad bought her flat. She was very interested in you and we stayed in touch. She had been managing a shop in the High Street until recently but she was happy to leave it behind and try something different.

Challenging, she says, but possibly more rewarding.

Over the summer, she has familiarised herself with your writing technique and has developed the confidence to write with you over more sustained periods. It is hard work for you, and I find myself continually humbled by the sheer determination and effort involved. But the result is that now, whenever you are in school, you will be able to communicate and record your thoughts, ideas, needs, feelings, anything. You can answer questions in class, you can even ask questions. If you are uncomfortable or unwell, there is someone on hand at all times to help you.

Within a matter of weeks, this new arrangement has proved an undoubted success and I can only wonder how miserable it must have been for you in school in the past. You are currently spending much of your school day in a standing frame, which enables you to write almost the whole time. You are very happy with this whole new way of working and you are starting to really enjoy your time in school.

159

So now the stories start getting back to me.

It seems that almost every day your assistant has a new anecdote about you. Each one more incredible than the last. The amazing answer you wrote in maths, the little poem you wrote about the pyramids, your interest in Queen Elizabeth, the boy you've taken a shine to. And then there is mischief too, the fun, the little confidences you share with your assistant. The sly written asides during lessons. There seems to be a completeness now about your experience in school that is so heartening to witness. I am equally pleased to see that your intelligence seems to be now moving beyond a matter of faith and conjecture. Actually, I am told that your new class teacher thinks that you are one of his brightest pupils.

And then I learn about the games.

These are the games you have been playing ever since the start of term with your assistant and your speech therapist. One of the games is called the whisper game. Your assistant has to leave the room and while she's away your speech therapist will whisper a secret word to you. Then, when your assistant returns, you have to write the secret word with her; the word that only you know. The words are chosen fairly randomly; in the last session, it was 'ketchup'. You are very good at this game and always get the secret word right. Your speech therapist is very happy too. The whisper game, I quickly discover, is one of her ongoing methods of informal validation. It is proving beyond all doubt that it is you who is writing and that you are not being helped in any way.

And in conclusion?

Through this simple process of validation, slowly but surely, I believe we have stumbled upon the proof I have been so desperately searching for all this time. If the writing proves your intelligence and the validation proves the writing, then the intelligence is surely proven.

But there is more.

There are other means of validating your writing. Your tendency to extend your vocabulary by spelling words phonetically and your somewhat curious but consistent syntax is often a good indication. Apart from spelling daddi and mummi in your usual manner, you will always write for first person singular 'my' instead of 'I', as in 'my hungry'. This, you will subsequently explain, avoids any possible confusion between I, 'l' (lower case 'L') and the number 1. Actually I think it makes a lot of sense. You also capitalise the 'e' in yes. This sole use of capitals in your writing results from the first two letters of yes in your particular handwriting looking a bit like no. I imagine that this is a confusion that anyone would wish to avoid. There are a number of similar quirks and idiosyncrasies and, if someone attempts to write with you, assuming that no examples of your writing have been previously studied, looking out for these odd letters is often the easiest way of showing that it is all your own work. Beyond that, I think these examples of you adapting words show how well you recognise problems and set about solving them.

Then there is the story of the bangles.

Towards the end of your first term working with your assistant, I am shown another example of you working through a problem in your own unique way and finding its solution when we all go to Greenwich Market one afternoon. Now you're a bit older, I give you some pocket money each week and this week you have decided that you want to visit the jewellery stand and buy bangles. You have earlier stated that these are not for you but you want to buy them for your assistant. I notice that she already wears a couple but you insist you want to buy her some more. She is deeply moved by your generosity and I tell you that you are incredibly kind. This will happen again on a number of occasions and you eventually purchase quite a collection of bangles. You are keen that she wears them to school and naturally she is happy to oblige.

The subject is then all but forgotten until you are chatting to your speech therapist one day. She mentions the bangles and you explain that if your assistant wears bangles you can hear them jangling and you know she is not far away. You don't have enough physical movement to turn your head and look around you, and if you're in a standing frame or a wheelchair you can only see what is directly in front of you. This is the method that you have devised to reassure yourself that your help and assistance are nearby.

I just think it's a shame that your school doesn't give out gold stars for problem solving.

You are seven years old today and this will be your first birthday in our new house. But you are not a very happy girl.

Your birthday this year falls on a Sunday and despite the promise of the Sunday lunch you have requested later in the day and all kinds of great presents, you seem downhearted on what should be your special day. Your mother and I try to chat to you at various points throughout the day but you seem reluctant to discuss the matter beyond informing us that you are a 'bit sad'.

The day passes without further comment, crisis or incident but I remain curious about what might be responsible for such a shift in mood. It casts rather a cloud over the whole day. When you have gone to bed, I wade through the abandoned ruins of another birthday and attempt to tidy up the lounge. Then, as I am sifting through the pile of cards, I realise that the young chap in your class who you have rather a thing for, failed to send you a card. Or give you a card in school like your other classmates. A couple of months ago, he also conspicuously failed to send you a valentine card. You sent him a very nice one as I recall and I think that hurt you at the time. Perhaps you had really been expecting to receive something from him for your birthday and what we have seen today is simply your first brush with disappointment in love.

Ah, how I would so dearly love to be flippant about all this and tell you that he's just a typical bloke and you shouldn't worry about him; they are all quite frankly useless. But I don't

162

imagine that there is much, if any, comfort to be found today in such remarks.

I so hate to see you sad like this and I feel so helpless. Back pains, toothache and stiffness I can help with – I'm not so good with a broken heart. Faced with my utter inability to do or say anything to improve the situation, I resort to telling you the following day over breakfast that I understand your problem and appreciate what you're going through. You look thoroughly unconvinced at this assertion and I don't blame you. I suggest that we go to Bromley after school and spend some of your birthday tokens. It is a weak suggestion but the only one I can think of at the time.

So, after school, your assistant and I take you to Bromley for an hour or so to look around the shops. You don't seem particularly inspired by anything you see or by any of our suggestions. No videos, books or CDs spark your interest today. I am about to write the afternoon off as a bold, well-intentioned failure when your assistant puts a pen into your hand and, holding a small notebook, she asks you if you have seen anything today you would like to spend your vouchers on. Your answer is succinct and direct. It is also something that I would, given an infinite number of chances, never have guessed.

'want buy blues.'

A little puzzled, yet more than a little curious, we ask you if you mean blues as in blues music.

'yes.'

Rather than risk giving you anything further to be miserable about, I accede to this rather singular request. In a state of some bewilderment, we take you into the branch of HMV, where we find you a couple of cheap CDs. Their stock is by no means expansive but I select a various artists' compilation of electric blues and a collection of songs by Muddy Waters for you. Whilst mindful of spending money in vast amounts on what is probably a momentary whim, I feel that these should satisfy your sudden apparent need for blues music.

But it is not a momentary whim.

It is far from being a momentary whim.

I can't begin to guess what prompts this sudden urge, whether you feel that there is something in the music that matches your mood at this moment or if you just fancy listening to something a bit different for a change. But from this day forward you will become absolutely fanatical about the blues.

You listen to your CDs as soon as you get home and I notice that your mood suddenly seems to lift and you are altogether much happier. It is, of course, possible that this is just a coincidence but I prefer to think you knew precisely what you needed to cheer yourself up. I am not sure if this can also qualify as problem solving on some level but you have now broken the spell and the curse is lifted. At the very least, I suppose this is your very own sort of music therapy.

The following day after school you ask to listen to your blues again, and again this seems to really lift your spirits. You quickly show a preference for the Muddy Waters CD and it is not long before you inform me that you 'want more muddy'. This is the first time you have expressed such a strong interest in music (besides your brief Take That phase and slightly more enduring Oasis phase) and so, over the coming weeks and months I buy you some more Muddy Waters CDs. Over time, as your interest grows, you also start accumulating recordings by Howlin' Wolf, Sonny Boy Williamson, Jimmy Reed, John Lee Hooker and many others, and you amass quite an impressive collection.

For reasons I will never fully fathom, ones that will remain forever private and personal, you absolutely adore this music. You never weary of listening to it and over time it becomes a very important part of your life. Beyond that, it becomes part of who you are, an aspect of identity rather than a simple preference. Acting upon further requests, I get you a couple of books about the history of the blues and these enhance your experience of the music still further.

But the music is what matters most to you. Within a matter

of months, you develop a near evangelical devotion to Muddy Waters and, having decided that his best work was *Live at Newport* (and in particular 'I Feel so Good', your absolute favourite song of all time), you spread the word by regularly giving copies of this particular CD to the uninitiated as birthday and Christmas presents. His music, you say, makes you happy and no further qualification is needed.

Your new interest raises a few eyebrows at school but personally I'm delighted that you have found music that I will for all time regard as *your* music.

You are seven years and 98 days old and I notice that after returning from school this evening you once again seem a little miserable. I assume that you are simply tired and that an hour or so with Muddy will sort you out. Then, with little preamble and no ceremony, your mother, who has been writing with you in the other room, walks up to me and hands me a piece of paper on which you have just written: 'why my body no work?'

I knew that this would happen one day but I just assumed that day would be far off in the future, in your teens maybe. Time enough for me to have prepared myself, to work out what I am going to say. But you are an intelligent young lady, intelligence being the value placed on good questions as much as good answers, and I suppose this shouldn't come as too much of a surprise.

'why my body no work?'

The brutal honesty of these five words buries itself deep within my consciousness and I know that it is not possible for a person to live long enough to forget a moment like this.

Your mother insists that I am better at this sort of thing and suggests I talk to you. So I sit you on my lap and try to explain what happened to you during your birth and how your brain was starved of oxygen. I try and explain in simple terms that this means that you are unable to walk or stand or do the sort

165

of things with your body that other children can. This seems to be achieving very little and you seem, if anything, to be more miserable. Then I explain that I too had an accident a long time ago and I fractured my skull and, as a result of my accident, I am deaf in one ear. So part of me doesn't work either. This also fails to have the desired effect.

Then suddenly I am able to find the words I am looking for. I tell you that all the greatest things in human experience are felt with the heart or the mind. That is where our great defining moments occur. The things that we will look back on when we are older, the things that we will gain most comfort from, are those moments that are spiritually or emotionally enriching. I tell you that I think that not being able to feel or to love would be a far greater loss to me then not being able to walk. It is at this point in our conversation that I first notice a change in your expression.

I tell you that I realise what the world must seem like from the perspective of a permanent observer and it is very sad that your body doesn't work, but you are actually quite lucky that your brain is so clever. Because you can think and that is one of the greatest gifts of all. And sadly, there are many young girls and young boys who are not as fortunate.

Perhaps it's just better for you to be clever.

Then, despite having no experience in these matters, I briefly and rather awkwardly attempt to introduce a more spiritual aspect. You have always been quietly religious in your own way but whether you believe in the Judeo-Christian God or Allah or Krishna, you could believe that there is a purpose and a reason why your body doesn't work. Maybe a reason that is not yet apparent. Perhaps you have been chosen to, one day, do amazing things and to do these things you need to be especially clever. You need to develop your mind and not think about your body, and perhaps this is the way your God has chosen for you. Maybe you'll write wonderful poems or paint the most brilliant pictures. Or one day, just by your example, you will

166

make a difference to the lives of everyone you ever touch. You will remind people of what is possible in life, not to grieve for what is taken away but to appreciate and celebrate what remains.

As a final strategy, I tell you about people who are brilliant who also have bodies that don't work. The most obvious example is, of course, Stephen Hawking. I explain that Professor Hawking is the greatest scientist of our time and he is in a wheelchair and communicates with a computer because he is unable to talk. Yet without doubt, he is one of the cleverest people in the world.

Then, I put you in your chair and put a pen in your hand. I ask you if you feel better.

'yes.'

Then I ask you if you think you would be happier running around the place or being clever just the way you are. You think for a moment or two.

'clever.'

I pick you up and hug you.

The following day we take the train into town and visit the National Portrait Gallery. Although we have visited the gallery in the past, the sole purpose behind this trip is to take you to see the recent portrait of Stephen Hawking.

I push your wheelchair right in front of the portrait and you look at him intently for a long time. I sense again that a season is beginning as I become aware that that one has just ended.

You are fourteen years old today and this year everything about your birthday seems to be related to you being an artist. You are given new brushes, paints, books and DVDs about art. But for your main present I have set up a website for you. It is your online gallery and you will be able to show examples of your work, which we can update as you do more and the website will also enable you to sell your paintings.

The original plan was to have the domain name sophie-art.com or ssj-art.org or something fairly simple like that. But then something happened in your schoolroom fairly recently that changed all that.

You had been having a lesson about haiku and minimalist poetry and at its conclusion you were encouraged to write a short three-line poem on any topic that interested you. As a subject, perhaps not surprisingly, you chose art. You then wrote:

wet paint
putting dreams
on paper

This was something you just wrote hastily at the end of your lesson but it struck me immediately as an amazingly profound and apposite summary of your whole attitude towards painting.

Putting dreams on paper.

From that day forward I have never been able to look at one of your pictures without that fabulous expression dancing into my mind. sophie-art.com was quickly forgotten and I registered dreamsonpaper.com as your domain name.

I show you the website on your laptop and you seem delighted to see your work displayed like this. There are about 30 or 40 of your paintings on view and it's a fairly representative selection of your work over the past couple of years. I'm sure that it is heartening for you, as much as it is for me, to note how many pictures have SOLD written underneath them.

The following month we are in Paris again and, as you do from time to time, you spring something on me that I could never have foreseen. Sometimes you may see or hear something that sparks your interest and very often I can trace the source of a sudden enthusiasm. But there are times like today when I realise you must mull things over and think about things for a long time. A while ago another one of your main preoccupations was the lingering desire to 'swim in the sea'. Similarly, I don't know what had placed that idea in your mind. Eventually we were able to comply with that particular request although I must say you didn't seem over-impressed with the experience and have barely mentioned it subsequently.

This morning, you are having a chat with your stepmother when, apropos of nothing in particular, you announce that you would like to be confirmed! She queries this and you boldly reiterate your previous remark.

'yes want be confirmed.'

Beyond the fact that you have been doing comparative religion this term in your schoolroom, I have no idea what might have triggered this sudden desire. It might have been something you have been thinking about for a number of years and now you are 14 you have decided that you are old enough. I tell you that I think that it might be a really good idea and we should make enquiries when we are back in England.

I can take absolutely no credit for your religious awakening and I confess that, whilst being far from atheistic, I'm not a churchgoer and I lack any particular orthodox faith. As far as I can recall, my only slight contribution to your spiritual tendencies is that a few years ago at your request we wrote a prayer together. This prayer sort of grew and modified itself over a couple of months as you added bits but it remains our sole collaboration of this nature and I still say it with you every night.

THANK YOU GOD FOR EVERYTHING.
THANK YOU FOR LOVE.
THANK YOU FOR JESUS.
THANK YOU FOR LIFE.
PLEASE GOD HELP ME TO BE A BETTER FRIEND TO THOSE I LOVE
AND GUIDE ME AND HELP ME ALWAYS.
PLEASE GOD HELP ME TO UNDERSTAND MY PROBLEMS AND MY
DIFFICULTIES AND THAT MY BODY DOES NOT WORK.
PLEASE HELP ME TO APPRECIATE THAT WHILE NOTHING CAN

CHANGE THIS I CAN, BY USING THE SPECIAL SKILLS AND TALENTS
YOU'VE GIVEN ME, FIND A WAY TO GO BEYOND THIS.
IF MY BODY DOES NOT WORK HELP ME TO SURPASS THIS.
SO I CAN FIND MY PLACE IN YOUR PLAN AND MAKE A DIFFERENCE.
HELP ME PLEASE TO APPRECIATE THAT THE GREATEST GIFT OF ALL
IS THE GIFT OF LOVE.
ANY DAY IN WHICH THERE IS LOVE IS AN IMPORTANT DAY.
ANY LIFE IN WHICH THERE IS LOVE IS A VALUABLE AND FULFILLED
LIFE.
AMEN.

You are fourteen years and 21 days old and now that we are
back in England again, I contact our local vicar and he calls at
the house to have a chat with us. He seems keen to offer you
all the help you will need to prepare for your confirmation. His
attitude is refreshingly positive and he seems to take some delight
in being able to assist you. We have already discussed with your
tutor the possibility of including work towards your confirmation
as part of your curriculum in the next term. The vicar says that
he will be happy to make regular visits and talk to you. He can
also suggest topics for discussion. It all seems like a very workable
programme and you are happy with the outcome. You are most
taken with the vicar and it's easy to see why.

Alongside theology, your new term's timetable will concentrate
on maths and art. After some discussion, it has been finally
decided that you should aim to take GCSEs in these subjects
and it has been agreed that you should be encouraged to focus
your time and your energy on them. Your tutor and your
stepmother will continue the working pattern they have
established with you over the past year and prepare you for
the challenge that awaits about 18 months in the future.

After some searching, we eventually find an accommodating
school in Dover who are happy for you to sit your GCSEs there
as an external candidate. Not long after the start of the term,

we have a meeting with the staff at the school and we discuss the practical aspects to your candidature. They are co-operative and extremely helpful.

For both the maths and art GCSEs you will be accessed on coursework and two supervised exams. You will be allowed extra time to complete the actual exams but the papers can not be modified in any way to take account of your disabilities. Obviously you can't use a protractor or a set square but sadly you will just have to lose marks on those questions when they are required. I also learn today that a person who acts as a support assistant in an exam situation is known as a 'scribe', which I rather like. The supervised exams will take place behind closed doors and under strict conditions; you will be scrutinised every minute by an independent invigilator to ensure that you receive no help. I have no worries in this regard but the truth of the matter is that I'd honestly rather you failed on your own merits than passed with assistance.

I would be so proud of you anyway.

As we are preparing to leave, I tell them that you might be a fairly special case but I'm sure you are far from a unique one. Again, it would seem, I am quite mistaken in this. My error is swiftly corrected. As far as the school is concerned, no pupil with your range of difficulties has ever sat a GCSE in a core academic subject like maths. They insist that it would be an extraordinary achievement.

This remark lingers with me and, all the way back to Canterbury, I wrestle with my conscience. I start to worry that I might be pushing you too hard to achieve something that is evidently so far beyond you. Not for the first time I worry that I'm forcing you to pursue an objective or a dream that is mine as much as it is yours.

I think I worry that I'm urging you to fight my battles for me and provide me with my proof. But I sense that our lives are now moving forward, shifting in emphasis once more and as a new season now begins so another has just ended.

171

Fifth Season

In Which There is Love

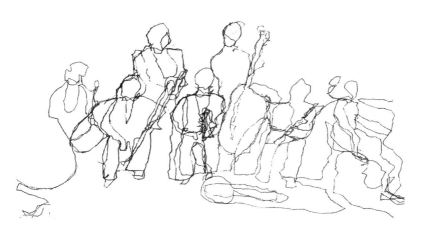

You are seven years and 177 days old and you spend a couple of days in Paris. Although this is not your very first trip abroad – you accompanied your Rimbaud-fixated father on a trip to Charleville near the French–Belgian border earlier in the year – this is the first time you have visited the French capital.

Your mother has opted out of this trip, as indeed she will opt out of many trips in the future and, instead, your assistant accompanies us. Taking on a more orthodox caring role, she has been away with us a number of times in the past when your mother and I have taken short holidays with you in Oxford and Brighton and such places.

You have enjoyed all your trips away in the past but this visit to Paris, which has been arranged hastily during your half-term break, will be different; it will turn out to be a most significant event in your life.

We take the Eurostar from Waterloo station and arrive in Paris in the middle of the afternoon. Our hotel is near the river on the Right Bank just off Rue de Rivoli, and after we've unpacked and you've finished your supper, we go out for a stroll. We wander up as far as the Louvre and back and we just soak up some of the atmosphere.

You are smiling when you go to sleep and you are smiling when you get up the next morning.

Over the next three days we walk miles and miles and do all the typical tourist things. We visit the Musée Picasso ('best museum in the world'), The Louvre, St-Germain-des-Prés, Les Deux Magots, Café de Flore, Place Vendôme and more cafés than I can remember. I have never seen you so happy, you seem to have this wonderful expression on your face virtually the whole time. You absolutely adore the place.

175

At the end of our long first day, your assistant puts a pen in your hand and we ask you what you have enjoyed about your day. By way of an answer you write for the very first time the four words that you will continue to write over and over again during the next four years.

'want live in paris.'

We also take you to Les Galeries Lafayette, which is one of the city's most famous department stores, and we buy you a couple of new items for your wardrobe. This visit coincides with your emerging interest in clothes and you take a great delight in selecting a couple of beautiful tops by agnès b. This actually is the start of a trend that will continue and, from this day forward, you will frequently insist upon only buying clothes by French designers whenever you are in France.

At this point in your life, rather like your continuing love of the blues, your clothes have become another very important aspect to your idea of yourself. It is a period in your life best exemplified by your decision to christen your two goldfish Emporio and Armani. Over the months you have become the owner of some fabulous individual pieces by various designers and you seem to love showing them off at every possible opportunity. If this is little more than an expression of vanity, then I am delighted that someone with your range of problems has found the means by which such a vanity can be expressed.

But whenever I think of you in some amazing outfit or another, I also like to think that on some level there is an element of defiance to it, a way of confounding expectation – so what if my body doesn't work – look at me, I can still be beautiful. And I am.

Our last morning in Paris passes in the blink of an eye and before we know it we are on the Eurostar heading back to Waterloo. All the way home you seem sad and the following day you only perk up when I get the photos of our trip developed. Together we spend a couple of hours putting them in a scrapbook. Naturally, I let you write the captions.

'want live in paris.'

Too often a parent's role involves taking all the magic and the dreams away from their children. But my parents never did that to me and I'm not going to do it to you either. I tell you that I think it's a wonderful idea and we should think very seriously about it.

One of the photos we took in Paris and which is now pasted into our album is a rather posed vignette of you and I sitting in Café de Flore. We are both looking directly at the camera and I am holding an advance copy of my second novel, which is to be published at the start of the new year. I began working on it before you started school and so I consider it to be a project that we briefly shared. It seemed therefore appropriate that I should dedicate the finished work to you.

A couple of months later the book is published as planned but what happens next takes me completely by surprise.

In drumming up publicity for the new novel, my publishers mention almost in passing the story of you first developing an awareness of writing whilst sitting on my lap at the computer while I typed. Suddenly everyone seems to want to know about you and me and our story. For about three weeks or so, we are the focus of considerable press and media attention. We are featured nationally in the broadsheets, the tabloids and magazines and on radio and TV. As may have been expected, nobody is all that interested in my novel but everyone is fascinated by our story, which, I keep reminding people, is your story. I just consider myself fortunate to have been part of it.

It is an extraordinary period in our lives. One weekend, a thousand word piece I have hastily written about us is featured in the Independent. This, however, is fairly overshadowed the following weekend when you are the subject of The Guardian Questionnaire! They have submitted a list of questions to us earlier in the week and you answer them over a couple of days with your assistant. You express a certain reticence about this

177

whole venture at first but change your mind upon being told that John Lee Hooker had recently been featured.

You answer most of the questions that I think are appropriate for a seven-year-old girl and you give a very fair account of yourself. Amongst other things, you say that you want to live in Paris, that your favourite fantasy is to meet Muddy Waters and you'd like to be remembered as someone who made a difference.

In answer to the question that enquires who is the greatest love of your life you reply 'my daddi'. While I publicly make a point of commenting that you are only seven and you are just a fairly typical daddy's girl, I am naturally delighted beyond words by your answer.

The theme that is constant throughout this and all the other articles at this time is that they refrain from lapsing into pity or sympathy. Indeed, they concentrate on your talents and your abilities and the tone is invariably positive, and most pieces conclude with an optimistic look towards the future.

You return to school the following week and it is generally agreed that your first brush with celebrity has had no noticeably adverse effects on you.

You are eight years old and this year your birthday is celebrated a couple of weeks shy of the actual date. Your special day is actually ten days early this year. I suppose it is a stage in development when instead of desiring objects and items for a birthday, a person begins to desire experience. I don't know at what age this usually occurs but this birthday has definitely marked your own personal transition.

You are still so passionate about the blues and for months now when asked what you would like for your birthday you have simply repeated that you want to visit the Mississippi Delta and see where Muddy Waters came from. It is explained that the southern states of the USA are such a long way away and it would involve being on a plane for ten hours or so but still you insist you want to go.

Initially, it was such a mad idea, but somehow over the weeks it becomes an increasingly appealing one and I begin to believe that such a trip might well be possible. I think it is the fear of simply becoming another person, just like all the others, who tells you that you cannot do something. I will not allow myself to become one of those well-meaning people who feel that it is their duty to place obstacles in your way. Or maybe it is simply that great roar of defiance again.

Who says you can't go?

It is a young lady's birthday after all.

So, on a fine spring morning you and I and your fearless assistant board an American Airlines flight at Heathrow and set out for Blues Country. Naturally, I have been worried for weeks about how you will cope with a long-haul flight like this but there is not the slightest problem. Your heart is obviously so set on this trip that you simply cope with any discomfort you experience. You are smiling and uncomplaining throughout and a delight to travel with. When we touch down in Memphis airport it is as though you have been taking the same flight for years.

We are staying in the famous Peabody Hotel, only a stone's throw away from the legendary Beale Street, and after checking in, even though we are tired from our trip, you insist that we take a quick stroll. There is a blues band playing on a street corner and you are in your element, and the moment I see the expression on your face I know we were right to make this trip.

Everyone we meet seems really interested in your story; for once disability is not the issue and people seem genuinely delighted that a young English girl, a few weeks shy of her eighth birthday, is such a devoted blues fan. At the various clubs and music shops along Beale Street, people make such a fuss of you and shower you with freebies. We watch a blues band playing at B.B. King's club and, for the benefit of all the

179

physiotherapists back home, I video record you sitting on your assistant's lap moving and dancing to the music. You can't walk, you can't talk, but you can't half boogie! Seriously, for someone who has such limited movement, it's an impressive and virtually unprecedented display and it remains one of the highlights of the trip.

However, the following day probably qualifies as your own particular highpoint. In fact, you will write at its conclusion that it was the 'best day ever'. We hire a car for the day and head south out of Memphis on Highway 61. Our trip takes us across the Tennessee border and into Mississippi and the town of Clarksdale about 70 miles away. For the duration you sit calmly in the back seat with your seat-belt on and generally behave like the seasoned traveller you are so rapidly becoming. After visiting the Delta Blues Museum in Clarksdale, where you make even more friends, we get back in the car and, following the precise directions given to us at the museum, we drive a few miles to the north-west of Clarksdale. We follow a few dusty roads until we reach our destination. Stovall's Plantation and the site of the wooden shack, which was home to the young Muddy Waters back in the 1930s.

We take you out of the car and we have a look around and you are so happy to be here. It is a quiet, fairly desolate, place and, although extremely atmospheric, there is very little to actually see. But the look on your face confirms that this means so much to you.

It strikes me at this moment that there are probably very few eight-year-olds who'll be celebrating their birthdays in a similar fashion this year. But there is no doubt that this is the perfect day for you. You are so much your own person nowadays and, beyond simply being your birthday, this trip is a celebration of that fact. We return to Memphis where we buy you some Muddy Waters CDs (which you don't already own) to commemorate the day.

The following day it rains mercilessly and we visit the National

Civil Rights Museum. It is a marvellous and inspirational place and it has a deep effect on you. You learn about Martin Luther King and his struggle and at the end of the day I ask you how it made you feel. At this point, I confess I make the thankfully rare mistake of thinking how you might respond. I imagine you writing 'sad' or that you found it 'upsetting' or 'moving'. I am therefore surprised but oddly uplifted when you write 'strong'.

After flying to Dallas, we return to England the following day and, while you cope equally well with the journey home, I suspect that part of you is still lost somewhere in Mississippi.

You are eight years and 55 days old when your assistant informs me that your new class teacher would like a word with me. I am assured it is nothing to be concerned about and it is simply an informal chat. Intrigued rather than worried, I contact the school and arrange an appointment for the following day. Having satisfied myself that it is not a serious issue, I speculate on alternatives. Maybe it's about the couple of school days you missed at the start of our USA trip, or perhaps I've fallen behind with your dinner money again.

But your new teacher doesn't want to talk about anything of that nature. In fact he opens the proceedings by informing me that you are very intelligent. The two of us are sitting alone in an empty classroom at the end of the school day. You are one smart cookie, he reaffirms, as though the point might be better made in the vernacular. I have absolutely no idea where this is leading and so I simply nod my agreement.

He goes on to tell me that in a class of children with very mixed abilities there are inevitably those who get left behind, who simply cannot cope with the work. But there are also pupils who are bright and they can sometimes suffer from being under-stimulated. They enjoy the work but they are not being pushed as hard as they might be. At this point I realise that he is talking about you. He is basically telling me that he can't give you the time that he feels you may need. He explains that he can't exclude the rest of the class and spend the necessary time with you to get the best out of you. Taken aback and overwhelmed by his honesty, I find that I am lacking the vocabulary to make any suitable response.

He then tells me that someone with your range of physical problems combined with your level of intelligence is not uncommon but it does present problems to a teacher; particularly in a class with a dozen other pupils. He shows me some of the work you have been doing in school this term and examples of the writing you have done with him and then, answering my next unspoken question, he suggests that if you could work with a personal tutor, naturally alongside your assistant, you would have the sort of attention that a class teacher can not provide. You would benefit from the level of scrutiny, an ability-based curriculum and the constant stimulation. He suggests that I look into it as maybe an additional after-school activity or for one day a week. Just to see how well you cope in a situation like that. Obviously, he adds, there is no guarantee that it will work, you may find it too much for you but it would surely be worth trying. Naturally, the school doesn't have those sorts of resources available and a tutor would have to be found in the private sector. I tell him that I didn't think that there would be many special needs private tutors in the phone book. 'Who said anything,' he asks without missing a beat, 'about special needs?'

I am so used to being on the defensive in situations just like this one; I seem only able to respond to doubt, denial, obstruction and negativity. I take a sort of pride from the fact that I've actually become rather good at it over the years. But when someone speaks of you like this in such glowing terms I am reduced to mumbling gratitude and fairly dim-witted questions. The last of which he replies to by informing me that he doesn't actually know of one and there is no one he could actually recommend. He is simply alerting me to the possible benefits.

182

I thank him again and then I thank him again and then I leave.

At roughly this point in your life I begin to observe what I perceive to be your mother's slow abdication of responsibility. You write regularly in school with various people about the problems that you have with your mother, and relations between the two of you have soured over recent months. I try to remain impartial and I refuse to take sides – not simply out of my usual cowardice but because it is hard to be utterly sympathetic with either viewpoint. During one particular heated exchange with your mother, the accusation is made that there have been three people in this marriage since the day you were born. Harsh words but ones that are difficult to refute, I suppose.

Guilty as charged.

But the idea of employing a tutor is discussed at some length over the next few days and your mother agrees in principle that it might be a worthwhile experiment. I contact a few local agencies and scour the local press, looking for available tutors. I call a few numbers and chat to a couple of them. A number of them seem keen and interested until I explain the specifics of the work involved, after which their tones become noticeably more reticent. Eventually I manage to speak to one woman who sounds as though she might be perfect for the job. She lives locally and I invite her to call in the following day so she can meet you.

She arrives at exactly the appointed time and we make small talk while I make her a cup of tea. She has a rather foreboding and forthright manner, yet there is something reassuringly scholarly about her and she manages to remind me of all my old teachers. I explain what the work would involve and she seems to grasp fairly quickly what is required. She confesses that her rather disciplined approach might nowadays be regarded as fairly antiquated but she would initially concentrate on the basics: multiplication tables and good fundamental maths skills and spelling. In my mind I have already given her the job but I take her into the large spare room on our ground floor, which will, from today and for the next few years serve as your first schoolroom. I introduce her to you and your assistant and she makes a point of talking directly to you. She explains roughly what sort of work she would like to do with you and that she thinks that the two of you might do some great things together. I make fleeting eye contact with your assistant and the matter is decided.

We are going to try a whole day for a couple of weeks and see how we get on.

You are eight years and 81 days old and you have your first home lesson with your first tutor. In the past week I have put a couple of tables and a desk in the schoolroom and put posters and charts on the wall so that it is a good working environment for you. It is also separate and distinct from the rest of the house and you will only ever use the room when you are having a lesson.

Your first lesson, I am told, went reasonably well, and over these first few weeks a whole new system of working begins to take shape. Your assistant and your first tutor work very much as a team, coming up with new ideas for every lesson. One of their first suggestions, which I put into practice immediately, is to print out your multiplication tables and pin them on the wall next to your bed. You can study these at your leisure when you are waking up or drifting off to sleep. When you have been tested on your three times table and get the answers right, the chart by your bed is taken down and replaced with the four times table and so on. The process continues in this fashion until you know all your tables. Similarly, words that you fail to get right in spelling tests are placed next to your bed for you to mentally digest. It is a fairly simple procedure but the results speak for themselves; within a matter of months I am able to inform your school that you have now been tested thoroughly and you know all your tables.

It is from this moment onwards that your level of achievement at home and at school become radically different. There will never again be even a suggestion of equivalence.

The school will, however, continue to set your targets for you. Your maths target now is to be able to use the correct formula to calculate area.

As the weeks pass, I contact your solicitor and am given some funds to help further furnish your schoolroom. We buy teaching aids, a computer and various bits of equipment, and ultimately your schoolroom becomes its own little self-contained primary school. You continue to express delight with the new arrangement and look forward to Fridays – your 'best school day'. Maybe it's the attention, the level of stimulation or the chance it affords you to show what you can do but the work you are doing at home continues to surpass everyone's expectations. I can only express delight that it is working so well. Hardly a month goes by without either your assistant or your first tutor devising a new idea that they would like to try with you.

The boldest of these is presented to me one Friday morning when I am summoned to your schoolroom. They have been discussing a new project with you and would like my opinion. Having discovered that your maths skills are well above average for your age, it has been generally agreed that you should now be concentrating on English. So, the bold plan is that you begin studying a children's classic book. Maybe a Dickens or *The Railway Children*. I think that it is a great idea and, while you are less than enthusiastic about the project, you eventually allow yourself to be persuaded. You are allowed to choose the book you want to study and after some consideration you decide on *The Secret Garden*.

This seemingly innocent choice will transpire to have been one of your most important decisions.

Over the next few months you become completely engrossed in the book. Something in the story evidently touches you on some fundamental level. There is, of course, the vaguely New Age-ish subtext of the story; the characters are each ultimately redeemed and healed by an understanding and appreciation of the natural world. But you absolutely love the story. Each Friday a chapter or two is read to you and you are then asked questions about the characters and the plot and how your attitude is changing as the story unfolds.

You are enjoying the book so much that you want to devote your entire school day to it and, in a display of truculence that will become all too familiar over the years, you refuse to do any other work in your schoolroom. No science, history or geography and no possible way to get you to put your maths skills to calculate area. I attempt to reason with you but it's quite futile. Besides, what does 'well-balanced timetable' mean to an eight-year-old? Particularly one who I suspect is smart enough to understand that she is, albeit indirectly, paying for these lessons. All I can suggest is that the project is continued, and as soon as the book is finished, you go on to something else.

The following Friday morning, my presence is once again required in the schoolroom. There is not a problem as such; I am just being informed at your request that you want your own secret garden. We actually have a fairly small garden at the rear of the house; it's not particularly secret, it's just rather nondescript. Actually, in truth, it's just not very nice and we rarely venture there. Apparently, you want to make a real garden for yourself out there, you want to redesign it, you want to cultivate borders and plant flowers, you want to paint fences and you want a lawn where you can lie in the summer.

I say that it might be a nice idea but I wonder if this is something that should be done at home, by which I mean not in the schoolroom. But your assistant and first tutor are ahead of me. They think the idea of working on your garden would be a great way of getting you back into maths and science again. I can't immediately see any connection but I bow to their greater experience and judgement. Even by the high standards you have set for yourself so far, what actually happens in the following few months is quite extraordinary. It seems that your first tutor was right.

Commencing the following Friday and working on your computer with hastily purchased 3D Garden Planner software, you begin to write down your ideas for your new garden. Your first tutor and assistant point out to me at lunchtime that this is the first time that you have used scaling skills and they are both delighted. But they have something else planned for the afternoon. Turning your attention to the issue of painting the fence and how much paint will be required, they manage to explain very easily to you the whole concept of area and the calculations involved. By the end of the afternoon you are calculating area with relative ease.

Maths sneaks into your day in the schoolroom again the following week when you are given a strict budget and told to cost the work on your garden very carefully. You seem quite delighted to do this; you are, of course, aware that you are doing maths but, rather than regarding it as simply an abstract mental exercise, maybe you now appreciate that it can also serve some practical purpose.

On your behalf, I engage the services of a gardener and, by the time he gets around to planting the flowers and vegetables you have requested, you are learning about different environments, different soils and the difference between acid and alkaline. You then have a day looking at life cycles, pollination, irrigation, photosynthesis and green issues.

This quite remarkable term continues in this fashion for a few more weeks. Your interest in your subject, your achievements and your workload all increase out of all proportion during this time. I keep the school regularly updated with what you have been doing and they can hardly believe what I am telling them.

Drawing on her experience, when project-based work was a vital part of primary teaching, your first tutor is convinced that this method is not simply the best way to teach you, it is quite possibly the only way.

The work on your beautiful garden is completed and *The Secret Garden* project concludes with you writing a poem about your new garden. It is a place where you find the magic in your life and where 'much happiness grows'.

We are not aware of it but we have just established a method of teaching that will take you all the way as far as your GCSEs and beyond.

You are fifteen years old today and you have been whisked away from your GCSE coursework and confirmation classes to celebrate your birthday in the French Quarter in New Orleans. Having famously failed to visit it once in the past, it is good to finally make its acquaintance.

Over the past couple of years your wanderlust has been mainly satisfied by shuffling back and forth between Canterbury and Paris. Recently, however, you have expressed the desire to see some more of the world. You wanted to go abroad for your birthday so we thought we'd retrace our footsteps and try New Orleans again. We have come as a larger party this time and we are accompanied by your stepmother, your grandma and your tutor.

Again I confess I have all my usual reservations about the actual journey but, as you have done in the past, you cope admirably with the ten-hour flight.

I wasn't really sure how you would feel revisiting the States, after all it's been seven years since our Memphis trip and this one feels like a sort of bookend to that first visit. I needn't have worried as you have a wonderful time. I don't know if it is the sheer joy of the place or the delight of travelling again but this birthday is a particularly happy one for you. I suppose

I should point out that you don't always respond so favourably to the places we visit. We have visited Venice and Amsterdam at various points in the past, both of which you enjoyed but you have never expressed the slightest desire to return.

At the end of our first day, you write that the French Quarter reminds you of Paris and, while that might sound like a fairly glib comment, there is a great deal of truth in this remark. Indeed, there is a very similar atmosphere to the place and, reluctantly at first, I fall under its spell too; New Orleans, like Paris, is one of the few places I have visited that is truly *l'égal de mes rêves*. You quickly submerge yourself in its history and culture. While not in its strictest sense a blues town in your mind like Memphis, it has its own particular musical story to tell and you soon succumb. We take you to Congo Square, to Bourbon Street, to Armstrong Park, to the Jazz Museum, to the impressive New Orleans Museum of Art and we take a trip on the *Natchez*, the last operational Mississippi paddle steamer and, once again, you are treated with great dignity and courtesy by everyone you meet.

At one point during our visit you actually write (for only the second time in your life) that you want to live here and for a minute or two I wonder, over there in Paris at this moment, just how securely the Wishboat is anchored.

A measure of your affection for the place is the pictures you produce upon your return home. For weeks you draw and paint various street scenes from the photos we took of the French Quarter. You work and rework various views with tireless enthusiasm. The pictures, which I feel to be amongst your finest landscapes, are crammed with detail and colour, and the artist's love is evident in every line and brush stroke. Naturally, four months later, you are devastated by the news reports of Hurricane Katrina. It is as though a special friend you have just made has been hurt or is in trouble.

In the meantime you return to working towards your GCSEs. As your tutor and your stepmother still use the same teaching method with you that was evolved all those years ago, naturally they still rely heavily upon your input. Your input at this time is to simply insist that more art and travel be added to your weekly timetable. It is also around this time that your tutor begins working with you on the novels of Jane Austen. I don't know why I should be surprised by this – by now I shouldn't be surprised by anything you do – but you are utterly captivated by these books. Starting, naturally, with *Pride and Prejudice*, you eventually work your way through the six major novels; *Persuasion* being particularly popular. But *Pride and Prejudice* remains your favourite. On one occasion you notably abandon your usual representational style and actually produce a striking semi-cubist abstract drawing of Elizabeth Bennet in which you portray her with two distinct faces.

I suppose I'm secretly rather pleased to discover that you have such a romantic streak.

Something else occurs during a lesson around this time that also takes me by surprise but has notably less academic significance. As part of a lesson about media and advertising, you are studying a woman's magazine. You spend the lesson going through it page by page, examining the content of the articles and the placement of advertisements. You are then asked to write your opinion.

Your opinion consists of one word.

It is a well-known four-letter word.

This is the first time you have ever included a word of that nature in your vocabulary and, while your tutor is understandably hesitant in condoning its use, it is generally agreed that in this particular context it is probably a perfectly valid and apposite comment.

While this becomes a favourite anecdote for a while, we do, however, refrain from mentioning it to the vicar when he makes one of his fairly regular visits. Everything is now set for your confirmation and the vicar has been discussing with the bishop, who will take the service, the best way you can receive your first communion. They are obviously giving the matter a lot of thought. As the actual date draws near, the vicar, who has expressed the highest regard for your painting in the past, asks you if you will do a picture of the church where the confirmation will take place. This will then be used as a colour cover for the order of service pamphlet.

You are naturally quite delighted by this and commence work on the painting without delay. When painting landscapes you are still mainly working from photographs but on this occasion you actually do some work in the churchyard. Nowadays, the posture you most frequently adopt while painting is lying prone over a foam orthopaedic wedge. You have a few of these scattered around the place: both homes, your schoolroom and your grandma's house. Over the years you have found that a prone-lying posture gives your hands the greatest amount of freedom and movement. Also a foam wedge is relatively easy to transport and, on the afternoon in question, your tutor and I set you up on it in a nice leafy, secluded corner, where you can get a good view of the church and work on your picture.

You work very hard on this painting and even abandon a number of your initial attempts. For any number of reasons, this painting is obviously so important to you and you are determined to produce something rather special. The finished picture certainly justifies all the extra work you have put in. It is beautifully detailed and well composed; in fact it is perfect for its purpose. When you are happy with it, I scan the picture and give a copy to the vicar.

With your confirmation a week or so away, we spend a few days in Paris with a view to buying you a confirmation outfit. I want to buy you something special and suitable that you will wear for the service and not wear again thereafter. It is also the chance for me to make a tangible contribution to the day so I want you to feel that this is not just you and I shopping for clothes but that this is us doing something important. Eventually, in Les Galeries Lafayette we find you a beautiful two-piece white linen suit by Christian Lacroix. It's a wonderful little outfit and you look fabulous in it.

It is of course fairly obvious but it only strikes me when we are back in the apartment looking at the suit. At some point it occurs to me that I may get no nearer to being the father of the bride and helping you choose a wedding dress; that this is as close as we will ever get.

Maybe this is an important time for me too.

The day before the actual day of your confirmation, with some reluctance I finally accede to your request to have your hair cut very short. I'm fairly certain that it's an Audrey Hepburn thing but I'm sorry to see you lose your beautiful curls. However, I have to admit the new style does make you look more grown-up and I imagine this is the point of the exercise. You sleep badly that night, it might be a touch of what you call 'lady pains' but it's probably nerves or excitement.

The confirmation service is set for seven o'clock and it's a beautiful mild-July evening when we make our way to the church. I take your picture and have a quick word with you. I tell you again that I am so proud of you and that I really admire you for deciding to do this, to declare your faith and see it through to its conclusion. It is not just the haircut or the new outfit, there is something different about you today, something I am seeing for the first time. Hard to define precisely, but in your face and your manner there is a serenity about you this evening. It is an expression of complete involvement with this moment in your life, I see now that it matters to you in more ways than I could ever imagine. I also sense that there is a strength about you too tonight, a strength of conviction and of purpose.

Somebody hands me a copy of the order of service with your picture on the cover. It looks wonderful.

Every day, I think, but maybe just a little more this evening, I feel genuinely humbled and honoured that you are my daughter. If these words sound forced or awkward it is only because they are so seldom spoken out loud. Sorry.

The service, during which you are one of about a dozen people being confirmed, goes exactly according to plan; the vicar and the bishop's modifications to the service work perfectly. Your tutor, who reverts to being godmother for the occasion, and your godfather, recite your words on your behalf as planned and the whole service takes place in front of the altar steps to make allowances for your wheelchair.

The service concludes and we return home. You are asleep within the hour.

It was such an important day for you and the following day you show your gratitude in your own unique way. You ask me to find a frame for the original painting of the church and this you give to the vicar. Then to thank your tutor, who managed to successfully juggle her role with that of godmother throughout, you place in her keeping your beautiful white confirmation outfit. Both of these gestures, it should be said, are greatly appreciated.

You are fifteen years and 201 days old and we have a problem.

We have just returned from a long weekend in Cairo, where we took you to see the Great Pyramid at Giza and the Sphinx. For a few years now you have expressed the desire to visit Egypt and I thought it would be a nice little break for us. There may have been some subliminal connection with your confirmation but I am not completely convinced by this. Once again you are a perfectly well-behaved and ceaselessly co-operative travelling companion. Furthermore, you are, by your own admission, quite overwhelmed by the pyramids and I rate the holiday a great success.

Perhaps it was too successful. Because not only do you start suggesting that you immediately begin studying travel as a part of your school timetable, you also, upon your return, categorically refuse to do maths. You will not write a single thing during lessons other than to reiterate that you do not have the slightest intention of doing maths ever again.

'no maths.'

Your GCSE is a matter of six months away but you have decided that you want nothing to do with it. It was the one academic subject at which you could really shine but, as I have discovered in the past, you can be so incredibly stubborn once your mind has been made up. I can find no way of reasoning with you.

'hate maths.'

You are reasonably content and happy the rest of the time – you are just adamant that you will never do maths again. Your tutor and your stepmother are both of the opinion that this might be a fairly obvious expression of traditional teenage rebellion and, as such, there is probably very little we can do to remedy the situation. They ask me how I think they should proceed with your schooling and, truthfully, I tell them that I have no idea. We try reasoning with you in so many ways, we are not even above resorting to the *you have this gift and God has given you this gift, etc., etc.'* ploy. We explain that this is your chance to really make a difference and to show anyone whose body doesn't work that so much is still possible.

'no maths.'

I realise that we are getting nowhere. Part of me wonders if it might be the fear of failure, an affliction that is common to virtually all pupils cowering in the shadows of their GCSEs. At one point you write something that partially confirms this and chills me to my very core.

'too much pressure.'

At this moment I instantly cease to question your reasons for abandoning maths and predictably I begin to doubt once more my own motives for pushing you towards this sort of accreditation in the first place.

Is it really to prove you right?

Or is it just to prove me right?

But before I can reach any kind of conclusion, your stepmother has another suggestion.

Having noticed that you seem to suffer quite badly with crampy PMS symptoms and often show signs of quite evident mood swings, what you term your 'lady sad', she wonders if your recent problems might be related in some way. In a lesson you recently had about periods and various arising symptoms, with your customary flair you likened your own experience to having a 'messy head'. Your stepmother firmly believes that this is related to your refusal to do maths. I confess that my first instinct is to disregard the suggestion, it sounds too simple, too obvious and things are so rarely like that, particularly things that have anything to do with you. But faced with no real alternative solution, I agree that it might be worth investigating.

After doing some research, your stepmother recommends that we try to introduce omega oil into your diet. Apparently it is just added to your evening savoury meal and this, she assures me, will have the desired effect. Again, my immediate reaction does tend towards the cynical but I concede that there is no harm in trying. So we take a trip to our local health and whole food shop and buy a big bottle of omega oil. It is apparently tasteless in food but, before adding it to your supper for the first time, I explain to you that I'm adding something that might help with the 'lady sad'.

As part of a strict regime now, we continue to do this every evening for a week or so, during which time the subject of maths is not even referred to in your schoolroom. Your tutor and your stepmother have agreed not to mention it and you seem in no hurry to bring the subject up.

Then one morning the theory is put to the test: with little or no ceremony, half-way through your morning session, a question is sneaked into your lesson. The topic under discussion is the imminent January sales in the big Paris department stores. Your stepmother confesses that when confronted with a price tag that says something like 300 euros minus 40%, which is a fairly common practice in the sales, she is utterly dumbfounded.

Your tutor agrees and asks you if you think that would be a bargain.

Instead of offering your opinion you simply write '180'.

They try again and ask you if a price tag of 250 euros reduced by 30% is worth having.

Again you write '175'.

This continues for the rest of the morning and in the afternoon you are back doing fractions again. At some point during the afternoon, I receive a phone call from your tutor informing me that the mathematician is back and a particularly dark period in your education comes to a welcome close. You return to your coursework and never again issue us with a 'no maths' ultimatum.

Over the years you have presented me with so many challenges, some are impossibly complicated. But sometimes, I'm now delighted to discover, the solution, like the one for a 'messy head', can be deceptively simple. It is never too late to learn an important lesson and omega oil will, from this point onwards, become a constant fixture of your daily diet.

You are sixteen years old and on the morning of your birthday you wake up in New York City. Your GCSE coursework is now completed and, after working so hard, I thought it might be nice to come away again for your birthday. In the past you have mentioned that you would like to visit New York and this seemed like the ideal opportunity.

We are staying at a hotel on 52nd Street, a short distance from Times Square, and after opening birthday cards and presents with you, we make our way to MoMA, where I keep a long standing promise to you.

All those years ago, when you first became interested in Picasso, we read about his art and his life and looked at examples of his work. One painting in particular, Les Demoiselles d'Avignon, had a particular significance, artistically and historically. Regarded by many as the single most important painting of the twentieth century, it stands as the first great masterpiece of cubism, abstraction and modernism.

When we visited Picasso's studio in Montmartre that time I explained that it was the actual place where he had painted *Les Demoiselles d'Avignon*, the painting that we had read so much about. Sadly, on that day, I had to tell you that the painting is not in Paris but at the Museum of Modern Art in New York. Then, on perhaps no more than a whim, I promised that one day I would take you there and you could see it for yourself.

And that day is today.

I push you in front of the painting and we remain there for a minute or two while you take it all in. Then I briefly sneak a few paces away and do something that you are not allowed to do in MoMA. I take a sly photograph of you. The picture will show you in profile dwarfed by the 8-foot canvas, totally absorbed in the painting, making your own connection, oblivious to all things, an artist lost in the wonder of art.

It has been another long trip but in that fleeting moment I know that it has all been worth it.

You paint a memorable, very atmospheric picture of a New York street scene upon our return but it is a subject you never again return to. From this and from a number of conversations, I conclude that while you thoroughly enjoyed the holiday and spending your birthday there, New York was not a place where you felt that great rush of emotional and spiritual empathy.

And so now you return to your daily lessons in the schoolroom. Admittedly you do so with a noticeable reluctance as a certain number of hours each week are now devoted to teaching you exam practice and what you can expect on the days you sit your GCSEs. Like any sixteen-year-old, this is not something you are greatly looking forward to. You are still doing ten minutes or so of mental maths every morning but no more than that. Your stepmother and your tutor consider this to be the wisest option – enough to keep you in practice but not enough to risk another rebellion from you. However, you have been promised faithfully that after you final maths GCSE exam you will never again have to do maths in any context.

I think the actual phrase in this case is an Uneasy Truce.

It's actually a shame as you have such a flair for numbers. But I suppose this qualifies as one of those moments that is common to all parents and not just those in my situation; that slight, perhaps selfish, disappointment that you feel as your child chooses or rejects something that you genuinely believe would be in their best interests.

In my parents' eyes, I must have done precisely the same thing a dozen times. Despite all appearances to the contrary, I wasn't being deliberately perverse and I am sure you aren't either. You are just growing tired of maths.

As the exam dates grow nearer, we hand in your art coursework. This consists of scrapbooks and sketchbooks of your work over the past year or so. In assembling your coursework there were times when we were forced to make allowances for the fact that you have sold so many of your finest pictures. I wondered if we might be allowed to submit scans of these works but when we contacted the school for their advice on this, I got the impression that this wasn't a problem they had encountered previously. But they advised against using scans.

Meanwhile you are currently working hard on preparing rough sketches for the picture you will soon produce under strict supervised exam conditions. Over the weeks your idea slowly reveals itself. It is planned to be simultaneously an interior and exterior view of a street in the French Quarter of New Orleans. Your plan is to paint a picture as two adjoining panels – the line dividing these panels is a wall that serves as a common feature to both. The interior panel features a dark corner of a bar where a rotund jazz pianist sits playing. Meanwhile, in the brightly lit street outside, Louis Armstrong as a young boy, leans his back against the wall and blows his cornet. He is watching a lady in all her period finery as she walks past. I am so impressed by this. You must have spent hours just thinking long and hard about this piece and even though it's an ambitious project, it is so clearly well conceived.

Over the years I have seen so much that convinces me that because you are unable to distract or entertain yourself physically, your brain takes over and is quite capable of keeping you occupied and stimulated indefinitely. A friend once compared this process to sitting in standing traffic completely bored and unoccupied. In such a situation it is not long before you are rescued from your surroundings by some sudden train of thought, something from your memory or your imagination, something that will take you away from the actual tedium of your predicament. The simple act of thinking at such times is beneficial and necessary. Out of boredom, or as part of a survival strategy, I really think your mind has developed its own highly tuned version of this particular skill.

You are never inactive – you are just busy thinking. And some of the time you are evidently thinking about ideas for paintings.

The night before your first supervised maths exam, I have a chat with you and tell you that you shouldn't worry and that you should just do your best. You reply to this by informing me that you are not worried, and in a strange way I take great comfort from this.

The following morning is warm and sunny and we take you to the school in Dover. We are met at the main door and I watch as you are quickly led away into a room accompanied by just your scribe and the invigilator.

The door is closed. You disappear from view and now I begin to wait.

You are nine years old today and for your birthday this year you request that we have a party in your new garden. It seems a very suitable way to mark the occasion and the weather for once is on our side. But beyond being a simple birthday celebration, today affords you the opportunity to officially unveil your new garden to family and friends. I have to say, and it is an opinion shared by all our guests, that it has been a remarkable transformation. The garden seems so alive now. One of the final additions to your overall scheme was a water feature and this was your suggestion to introduce an element of sound into your little sanctuary. I would never have thought of that and once again I am hugely impressed by the way you have conceptualised every aspect down to the last detail.

You invite your first tutor to your party and, with suitable ceremony, today marks the end of your work on *The Secret Garden*. It has been an incredible eight months or so but I think everyone is now ready to move on. A number of new topics are under discussion and the one that seems to be generating the most interest is Nelson Mandela.

Sticking fairly closely to the now established methods, your tutoring sessions continue to produce extraordinary results. It seems that almost every week I am sending something new into school for your teachers to see. The important thing is that you have established such a conscientious approach to your work in the schoolroom. You work diligently and consistently and look forward to your weekly sessions. In the first few months you used to tire in the afternoon but now you work at the same intensity all through the day.

Your first tutor has also been responsible for getting you involved with our local Brownie pack. It is something you really enjoy and every Wednesday evening you join your pack at the local village hall. I think it's good for you to mix with able-bodied girls your own age and they all seem delighted to have you as a friend. You won your first Brownie badge recently and you now have a collector's badge. You were awarded it, not surprisingly, on account of your Muddy Waters collection. That's my girl! For any number of reasons, I think the Brownies is actually very good for you.

The one issue that always crops up during discussions about you being taught at home is the one about you spending time with what is termed 'your peers'. Nowadays I counter this by saying you are a Brownie. But they are not referring to Brownies or artists or blues fans and the implication is quite clear. It is one to which I will take exception for years to come. *Your* peers, *your* people. Yes, you must spend time with *your* people! It is hardly the most inclusive of ideas and I find the implication of the term slightly offensive. Grouped together and neatly marginalised. It is an historically familiar idea but I will need a great deal of convincing before I consider it a beneficial one.

It is roughly around the time of your birthday that I begin to wonder if it might be worth you having two days of private tuition each week in your schoolroom. I mull this over for a few weeks and eventually call your solicitor to bring him up-to-date with your progress and enquire if the funds would be available to pay for two days tutoring.

The funding would not present a problem. However, it is pointed out to me that if you require a personal tutor in this manner, to enable you to reach your full academic potential, then you should not be paying for it yourself. If it can be shown that you need a tutor then it should be drafted into a new Statement of Special Educational Needs and the cost should be borne by our local authority and not be taken out of your funds. He also thinks that the authority should pay for your assistant, as her role is also fairly central to your education.

In principle, I agree with him completely, however, I am at this point blissfully unaware that I have just been handed my latest quest.

In pursuit of this new objective, I have a few meetings and make dozens of phone calls. The message becomes clear relatively quickly. The local authority will only fund personal tutors in the short-term for pupils who are convalescing. There is no precedent for funding a pupil in your situation and with your needs. That would appear to be the final word on the subject.

I convey this information to your solicitor who rather than concede defeat, suggests that we request that your Statement of Special Educational Needs is updated to include a tutor and we take your case to a tribunal. Towards this end, we will instruct an independent educational psychologist to observe you and build a case on your behalf. In the meantime you commence having two days in your schoolroom every week with your assistant, who goes wherever you go, and your first tutor.

At one of these sessions we first make the acquaintance of the independent educational psychologist who comes to observe you working. It is not a promising start. He is very dubious about the whole issue of 'facilitated writing'. I point out that after a couple of years of successful informal validation, the correct term, we have been told, is 'supported writing' but this doesn't impress him. He knows much more about this sort of thing, as is ever the case. He reiterates he can only make his assessment based on what he sees. As virtually every single one of your academic achievements is based on you writing, our whole case would appear to have just buried itself in the laboriously tilled soil of your new garden.

I don't know if I am upset or angry or just so weary of it all. I thought he had been instructed to work for you, to speak on your behalf, but it doesn't seem to be working that way. As though it might be considered some consolation, he explains that our local authority is unlikely to want a tribunal and would probably rather have the issue sorted before then.

He makes a few more visits over the next couple of months and remains cynical about the whole issue of your writing. I speak up in your defence, cautiously, as once again I catch myself slipping into the perceived role of deluded parent, and I have no doubt that he has probably met more than his fair share. In desperation, I even encourage him to actually write with you at one point and, while I can see recognisable letters in your usual style, he considers it 'inconclusive'.

One afternoon, I accompany him as he visits your school to

202

chat with your class teacher, various therapists and, in particular, your IT teacher. As we are driving, I raise the issue of compiling a report on you that fails to endorse your writing. Is such a report worth having? How can we claim that you need a tutor to stimulate you academically when all the evidence of your academic ability comes from your writing? He tells me that he intends to ignore the issue and work around it.

That afternoon I tour him around your school and introduce him to your teachers who show him examples of your work. I never see him again but true to his word, when I see a copy of his report a week or so later, he has indeed worked around the issue. In doing so, unlikely as it may seem, he might have provided us with another very different sort of validation. He makes no direct reference to your writing but concentrates instead on the very first work you did with your IT teacher. You were shown how to use your blinking response to select letters from a grid. It was a laborious process but at the end of the session you had selected the phrase: MUDDY WATERS BLUES SINGER.

Not a particularly surprising choice in itself but, as the educational psychologist concludes in his report, there is no possibility that you could have produced such a sequence of words accurately without already having the ability to write. More than the written evidence, in his mind, this better demonstrates your skills. Thus, from the most unlikely combination of sources, there is further validation, further proof.

The report, however, seems to achieve very little and our local authority seems unimpressed by it. Things grind to a halt once again and months go by. There is no further mention of a tribunal and one day I just grow tired of waiting. I do something that I have not done previously. I call the Directorate of Education directly and tell them I want to come in on my own for a meeting. No solicitors, no paperwork, just me on my own. Fine, they say, come in next week.

The day arrives and I make my way to the council buildings,

where I am shown into a room and introduced to two women from the Special Needs department. We sit on opposite sides of a big table and smile hopelessly at each other. Perhaps because I feel I have nothing to lose, I approach this meeting with notably more optimism than usual. Within a matter of minutes, I am delighted to discover that they seem equally keen to sort this issue out. Our man was right; they don't really want a tribunal and neither of us wants to waste any more time on further reports.

'What do you want exactly?'

'Well, what can you provide?'

The tone of the meeting is friendly and convivial, the spirit of negotiation and not confrontation, and eventually we are able to find a compromise. It is as simple and as easy as that. Beginning the following term, we will continue to fund your assistant (I actually prefer this arrangement as it means she will be able to work with you when you are not in school for any reason), but for one day a week, they will pay for a teacher to work with you in your schoolroom at home. Part of this new deal involves not using the word 'tutor', which is evidently a contentious term in this context. Instead, from this afternoon onwards, I must start saying 'off-site teaching support'.

I return home to tell you the news, it's a small victory but it is a victory nonetheless. Then I wonder, apart from those who are convalescing, just how many pupils have 'off-site teaching support' written into their Statements of Special Educational Needs.

Maybe it's not such a small victory after all.

You are nine years and 173 days old and we spend the weekend in Oxford. Meanwhile, back in London, your mother is moving out. This has been arranged so you are not forced to witness the actual spectacle. It is more than ironic that, in planning this weekend and sparing you the possible ordeal, your mother and I have recently managed to behave in a far more co-operative manner towards each other than at any point in the previous five years.

It is a debatable point if you would actually find it such an ordeal. Rightly or wrongly, justifiably or unjustifiably, you still display a certain animosity towards your mother. Regardless of your motives or your reasons, it is hard sometimes to be completely sympathetic. You can be quite a vituperative little soul when you put your mind to it. The whole rather dispiriting saga reached its apex earlier in the year when your school arranged for you to have regular weekly sessions with a specialist counsellor. This had been offered to you on account of what you had been writing about your mother with various members of the school staff fairly consistently over a number of months. In official documents the school refers to these incidents as 'perceived difficulties' with your mother, but they felt they had to take some kind of action.

The sessions seemed to be successful and at the end of one you return home with a letter you have drafted with your counsellor for your mother to read. I am not convinced that it has the desired, or indeed any, effect, but the sessions are discontinued shortly afterwards.

Good husband, bad husband, good father; the terms all seem arbitrary and relative and essentially meaningless. At least that's what I keep telling myself and I suppose it is just my way of avoiding the issue. Realistically, the odds were so stacked against your mother and I, a daughter born a month shy of her parents' first wedding anniversary. At that very moment lives were changed in ways that could never have been anticipated. On that same day I embarked on this great long journey with you and I could never quite get myself back home again. But the truth is I wouldn't have changed a single moment of it.

Father/daughter.

There has never been a single relationship in my life that has involved me so completely; neither has there been one that I have found so rewarding.

I imagine that there is no such thing as a simple separation but in this particular case the situation is possibly complicated by your dwindling relationship with your mother. Also, you are constantly defending and sticking up for me, and in your mother's eyes I imagine that this only serves to make matters worse.

We have a two-way split divided three ways.

You will continue to see your mother every other weekend but in the meantime my first decision, as a single parent, is to completely rearrange the house. The only room that is left untouched by this new regime is the schoolroom, and the week following your mother's exit you return to work with your usual enthusiasm.

Following the redrafting of your Statement to include the words 'off-site teaching support' we are now visited once a week by a teacher from your school. She is given targets for you by the school but works towards these by using the methods already established by your assistant and your first tutor. Your weekly timetable now consists of two full days in your schoolroom: one day with your first tutor and one day with the 'off-site teaching support', plus three days in school.

Coincidentally, the teacher coming from your school is South African by birth, so it seemed natural that you should study Nelson Mandela this term. You spend a number of weeks looking at the geography and history of South Africa but this time the subject doesn't seem to ignite your imagination. Both teacher and tutor try to engage your interest in the topic but over the weeks it seems in danger of becoming a futile exercise. I try to reason with you but it is to no avail.

Just as I'm beginning to wonder about all the great work on *The Secret Garden* and the virtues of involving the Director of Education, your assistant has a suggestion. Rather than concentrate on Nelson Mandela's struggles in South Africa, she thinks that maybe you could do some work on the broader issue of protest. At this point I think your team would be willing to try anything rather than concede defeat and waste the whole term.

So you spend a few sessions learning about the history of

protest and the means by which people protest. You look at everything from 'Strange Fruit' to *Guernica* and from Emily Pankhurst to Bob Dylan. Suddenly it happens again! With some relief, I am able to report that, with only a couple of weeks of the term remaining, this seems to really inspire you once again. You have always maintained that one of the greatest things that can be said of a person is that he or she made a difference and now you can see the whole idea of protest in this context.

Despite this last-minute surge of interest, I am worried that you have very little to show for this term's work, nothing to compare with all the amazing things that we were able to show off at the end of the time spent on *The Secret Garden*. Once again, your ever-resourceful assistant comes to our rescue with another idea. During the penultimate week of term, she asks you if there is anything you would like to protest about. And what form would you like your protest to take? As a sort of mental homework, you are asked to think about this for a few days and see what you can come up with.

'You really should come and see this!'

The following week you start your regular session with your first tutor and your assistant and within about half an hour I am summoned to the schoolroom in this manner.

'You have got to have a look at this!'

Apparently, you have been thinking very long and very hard about the task you were set and have conceived your protest in its entirety. In your mind the work is complete and it is simply a question of putting the ideas on paper.

The subject you have chosen for your protest is the lack of wheelchair access at our local railway station. The outward trips are fine but upon returning you have to be carried by two people up a long flight of stone steps. This is something you evidently feel very strongly about and it is a well-chosen and more than worthy target.

The medium you have chosen to voice your protest is, perhaps not surprisingly, a blues song.

What you have produced this morning and what I am now holding in my hand is one of the most remarkable pieces of work you have ever done. The four verses of lyrics you have written to your song absolutely astonish me. 'Sophie's Railroad Blues' follows precisely the repeated stanzas and rhyming schemes of the classic twelve bar blues. It's an extraordinary effort and so much thought must have gone into it. It is, in its own way, a perfect protest song; you detail your grievances succinctly and precisely over three verses and then conclude with:

If I can't get up the stairs then I'll just have to camp.
If I can't get up the stairs then I'll just have to camp.

You don't care or you would build me a ramp!

Your assistant and your first tutor are both equally stunned and in the space of half an hour you have produced something that I believe justifies the entire term's study. In the face of such an endeavour, it seems only fair that we should all do our bit too. So, borrowing a few ideas from the great Jimmy Reed, the following afternoon, I set your tune to music and record your song on a portastudio. I play the guitars and do a bit of harmonica but the vocal duties are taken by your assistant's daughter, who, it is generally agreed, sings your words brilliantly.

Once the song is recorded, I copy it on to a CD. Then, during the final home session of the term, the teacher from school drafts a letter with you. This letter is sent to our local MP and the local railway network and accompanies a CD of 'Sophie's Railroad Blues'. It lists your heartfelt criticisms and explains why you have written your protest song.

Eventually we get a reply from the railway network thanking you for taking the trouble to write, and this drab and dismal document sits in the folder of the term's work opposite the first draft of your lyrics.

I don't recall very much of the letter but your song still plays in my head to this day.

You are ten years old and we celebrate your birthday at the Bishopstock Blues Festival in Devon. It's another memorable birthday for you. I wrote to the organisers a few months ago and told them your story and how much you are a blues fan and asked if there was a chance you might be able to view some of the concert from backstage. The organisers were, I have to say, absolutely brilliant. I got a reply by e-mail virtually the next day. Not only did we all get free passes with unrestricted access for the whole weekend, they also arranged for you to meet the major blues artists who were performing there. Everyone is so incredibly pleasant to you and delighted that the blues means so much to you. At one point you are introduced to the legendary Taj Mahal who picks you up and talks to you. He signs a photo for you that says, 'To Sophie, loved meeting you...'

It is not a day you are likely to forget.

We return to London the following day and, after allowing us a day to recover, I accompany you into school the following morning as I've been told the new deputy head teacher of the school wants to see me. There has been a major change of staff at the school recently and there is now a new head teacher and deputy head. I have met the former on a couple of occasions, not always in the most cordial of situations, but this is the first time I will meet the latter.

'How do you like being a headmaster, then?'

The new deputy head is not one given to formal introductions it would seem. Somewhat bewildered by the enquiry, I smile awkwardly at her. She repeats her question.

'So, you're enjoying being a headmaster?'

She clarifies her enquiry by explaining that she has been hearing about the incredible things that you have been achieving

at home with your team and she tells me she is astonished b
the consistent quality of your work. As she rather flatteringl
invests me with some credit for its successes, she considers m
role to be an approximation of a headmaster. Furthermore, sh
is extremely interested in the actual method that has been use
to teach you.

I try to explain it as best I can, saying that the work ha
been topic-based and built up around your interests and abilitie
I falter at this point, as I've never really had to explain th
precise process before. It just sort of grew and developed an
it seemed to work. Whatever we have managed to stumbl
upon is evidently the best way of teaching you. If you show a
interest in something then the sessions can be built up aroun
that. These can spiral off in many directions but we can alway
find a way to work around the topic so your termly targets ar
always met.

I babble on hopelessly for a couple of minutes until th
deputy head has mercy on me. She informs me that sh
believes that there are a number of other pupils in the schoo
who could benefit from exactly the same kind of intensiv
personal tuition. She elaborates by saying that after years o
teaching in Special Schools, she has so often encountered pupi
very like you. Those that give every indication that there is s
much happening just below the surface. In a class of ten o
fifteen pupils there may be one, or possibly two, pupils tha
fulfil this criteria. It is so often just a question of finding th
way in.

She thinks there are currently about half a dozen pupils in
the school who could successfully be taught the way that yo
have been taught. It is not, she thinks, just a question of workin
with a personal tutor. It is more the way that you have bee
taught that is significant in your case.

Having no reason to disagree with her, I'm left with littl
alternative than to wholeheartedly concur.

Then, again with little preamble, she asks me another question

210

'How would you feel about setting up a schoolroom like the one you have at home right here in the school?'

I am stunned by the question but she goes on to elaborate further. A room could be found in the school, any room, it didn't really matter as long as it was big enough. The room would be fully equipped and self-contained and a number of carefully selected pupils each week could be taught in the same manner you have been taught. You could even have your full day of 'off-site teaching support' whilst remaining on the school premises. (This would certainly please your head teacher and anyone still firmly believing in the sanctity of peer groups.) She sounds terribly excited and it's hard not to share her enthusiasm.

I tell her I think it is a great idea.

She suggests that we start planning as soon as possible and lists a number of pupils that she believes could really excel with personal tuition. It will be a project that will run in the school but, in many ways, it will have its own agenda. She would like me to be involved, as she puts it, as a consultant. I tell her that I am flattered and that I would be delighted to help. For a moment, I think about you 'making a difference' and maybe this is precisely the sort of thing to which you have been referring all this time.

Beyond being a simple recognition of all the great work that you and your team have done, it seems such an important and worthwhile thing to do and I genuinely love the thought of passing on all we have learned.

She talks more about her ideas for the 'project' – the word has been chosen deliberately as it suggests that this is a method of teaching, rather than something attached to a particular school, and can be taught in any environment.

I can do very little aside from reiterate that I think that it is a marvellous idea. We shake hands and one of the most extraordinary meetings I have ever attended comes to a close. By the time I arrive back at home I have managed to digest the full significance of what is, if nothing else, such a positive acknowledgement and affirmation of all the great work you have done over the past year or so.

You are ten years and 83 days old and we are in Guy's Hospital where you are to undergo the scheduled major surgery to your back. This is an operation that has been long discussed and I have been dreading it from the moment it was first mentioned.

It is actually two full-day operations a week or so apart and we are to remain in hospital for the duration and for a week or so after. The purpose of these operations is to insert a couple of metal rods into your back that will fuse to your spine. This will prevent any further deterioration and curvature of the spine known as scoliosis. If the operation is a success it will mean that you will no longer have to wear your spinal brace and it should improve the quality of your life immeasurably.

Earlier this morning, before you are to have the first operation, I chat with the surgeon before you go down to theatre. He tells me that you are the smallest and youngest patient he has performed this operation on. I'm not sure that I want to hear this and I spend the day in a highly anxious state while I wait for news.

Unable to sit, or to read or to settle in any way, I occupy myself for a few uncountable hours walking around the grounds of the hospital. Unintentionally but possibly inevitably, I catch myself thinking back over the last ten years. Random images come to mind, not sorted by significance or chronology, just pages falling from a scrapbook. Me taking you out in your harness, your first music therapy lesson, writing 'you love me best' with me last night before you went to sleep, your garden, the lovely card the Brownies have made for you, that little smile that crosses your face the moment you hear Muddy Waters, the way you stretch in the mornings when I pick you up out of bed (have I ever told you how much I love that?). On and

n and while I wait for news, I feel as though everything is in
mbo again, suspended, paused and poised, an old familiar
eeling and suddenly I have no role, no history, no purpose and
o identity. I remain lost to time and the universe.

Later in the afternoon I get word that you are out of theatre
nd in the recovery room, and the blood begins to flow through
ny veins once again. After a few hours, I am allowed down to
ee you and find you distressed and rather angry about things.
ou can hardly be blamed under the circumstances, but it is
enerally thought to be a good idea to keep you in the recovery
oom rather than return you to the children's ward. I stay with
ou until someone suggests that it might be better for me if I
eturn to the ward and try to find somewhere I can grab a
ouple of hours sleep.

I don't appear to have the strength left to argue.

You are brought back on to the ward the following afternoon
nd seem exhausted after your ordeal. I put a pen in your hand
nd try to chat to you a bit but you fall asleep before we can
ven start.

The week between the two operations passes as slowly as
ime usually passes in hospitals. You pick up an infection at
ne point and are quite unwell with it. Your temperature is
vorryingly high and I wonder if this may delay the surgery but
'm told that they will go ahead anyway. The second operation
akes place as planned and I pass the time in a similar manner.
This one runs two hours over its scheduled time and when I
ee the surgeon walking through the doors of the children's
vard and heading towards me, I confess I begin to panic. I have
vritten and redrafted at least a dozen screenplays, each one
nore ghastly than the previous, before he even opens his mouth.

Actually he has come to tell me how well the operation went.
He is delighted with the result and how well you coped with
t. He says I can go and see you but before I leave he talks
gain about the long-term effects of your surgery. Due to the
usion of your spine, you will be unlikely to grow very much

213

more. You are a rather petite ten-year-old but you will neve be very much bigger. I was prepared for this as it had been discussed previously but I'd been trying not to think about i too much. For want of something to say I ask him what th rods are actually made of. He tells me that they are titaniur based.

I must have registered surprise at this because he goes on t clarify the matter.

'Well, they might have to last seventy years...'

At this precise moment I realise what the unspoken agend has been all this time, unspoken by everyone including me One of the greatest threats to life for someone with cerebra palsy derives from problems with the lungs. These problem invariably come about as a result of scoliosis and the constriction of the spine. Now, as a result of this surgery, this threat ha been significantly alleviated.

In this moment I realise that the goal is not just quality c life but also quantity.

In common with the general stereotype, I have found thi surgeon's manner a little brusque and insensitive at times bu at this moment I think I could quite happily hug him. I rush down to the recovery room to see you and find that you ar still peacefully asleep. I can't wait for you to wake up, I hav so much to tell you.

The following week, which coincides with the start of th summer holidays, we return home and you commence a mont or so of convalescence. Your assistant comes to spend som time with us and it is roughly around this point in our live that my relationship with her slips from the professional an into the personal. I am very careful that this has no advers effect on the equilibrium between the three of us. You ar actually delighted. I thought you would be; you have been suggesting that I marry her for at least three years.

So your assistant now gradually takes on the additional rol of stepmother, whilst continuing to function as your validate support worker. Her first task that combines both roles is the lengthy chat she has with you, during which you inform us that you want a cat. Your mother has recently acquired one and you have decided that you want our house 'be home for cat'. You go on to say that we will all love him and you have already settled on a name for him.

When you are questioned further upon this you write boldly and phonetically:

'bransun pical.'

I have no idea where or when you first picked up the phrase Branston Pickle but I must confess it is a perfect name for a cat. Again, it proves just how much of your surroundings you take in. How can I possibly refuse? So, I accede to your request and I buy you a beautiful white silver-tipped short-hair kitten from a local breeder. You are absolutely right, the house is so much better for having a cat about the place. Branston becomes a much-loved family pet and for the rest of the summer he is the perfect companion for a young lady recovering from her operation.

Whether or not Branston actually functions in any therapeutic way is debatable but nonetheless you are fully recovered by the start of term and you return to school.

It is a matter of a couple of days later when you have your first full day's session as part of the new project. The room they have found for you in the school would not have been anyone's first choice but there seems to be no alternative available. When I next meet the deputy head, she explains that she has encountered some resistance to her idea. She euphemistically refers to 'opposition from certain quarters' and I don't feel inclined to press the issue. However, the room where you and six other children will be taught according to the methods stumbled upon in your schoolroom remains a breakthrough. I am relieved and delighted that the first indications are that the other pupils are responding well and the results from the first few sessions are encouraging.

I promise the deputy head that I will continue to help promote the project. So far this has involved writing and printing pamphlet and designing letterheads but now I decide that it might be worth making a more public statement. I contact a journalist whose acquaintance I made a couple of years ago and tell her about you and the story of the project. She is very interested and we meet up a few days later. I tell her all about the schoolroom the great work you have done, the inadvertent discovery of a new teaching method and how your school now plans to follow your example by using the same principle to teach other pupils She tells me that she thinks it is a great story.

You and I have our pictures taken in the schoolroom but before she leaves I have arranged for her to have a short interview with you. She asks you a couple of questions and your stepmother is on hand so you are able to write your answers. You inform her that you enjoy this method of teaching because it enables you to 'work much harder'. When asked if you think that the project in school is going to make a difference to how pupils are taught, you reply 'big time'! Finally, she asks you how all this makes you feel. Your answer is 'proud, excited and very happy.' The following weekend the story is featured in *The Times*.

It is a positive and well-written article accompanied by two rather fine pictures of you and I. Of all the articles that have featured your story, this one has to be one of my personal favourites. I think that it is heartening that people are now aware of the great potential in this method of teaching and that hopefully children with similar problems to you will benefit in the future from what we have learned. But most of all I like the article because of its title:

SOPHIE AND THE SECRET GARDEN

I must confess it is only when I read the headline that I suddenly realise what an absolutely perfect metaphor this is and has been all along. Perfect in every possible respect and how we all managed to miss this I will never know! But it is an image that so perfectly encapsulates the sense of something being so alive and growing and developing, but imprisoned and shut in or simply obscured from view. It is hard work, a struggle if you like, but the rewards more than justify the quest and ultimately a great hidden truth is revealed.

You will always have a strong attachment to *The Secret Garden*, but from today, albeit belatedly, there is now a further dimension.

You are eleven years old and sadly this year your birthday is all but lost in the aftermath of an event three weeks ago. Having so enjoyed the trip to Memphis a couple of years ago, your stepmother and I thought it might be a good idea to try New Orleans this year. We plan the trip for the month of your birthday. Unfortunately, during the week we are planning to leave, my father is taken into hospital for his scheduled heart valve replacement operation. I visit him every day, and every day I wonder if we should be making this trip. He assures me that all will be fine and it's a fairly routine procedure nowadays.

So what actually transpires has a sickening, hideous inevitability.

The day before we fly, while you are at Brownies, I visit him in hospital and he informs me that his operation is also now scheduled for the following day. I tell him that most transatlantic planes have those credit card phones and I'll be able to call him after his operation.

It is the last thing I ever say to him.

The following day, whilst on an American Airlines flight 30,000 feet above Canada, I finally get through to the hospital. My father never regained consciousness and died during his operation. I break down and immediately start throwing up. It is too much to bear and I'm too far away. I think that by this point you have guessed what has happened but through my convulsive sobbing I manage to tell you that your grandad, my father, has died.

There is perfect silence for a moment and then you let out a piercing moaning sound. It is unlike any noise you have ever made before or since but it perfectly captures the moment and I love you for that. It is like our own private requiem.

Meanwhile, your stepmother has alerted the cabin crew to our problem and they immediately spring into action. They radio ahead to Fort Worth, where we are changing planes, and arrange to put us on a plane straight back to London. They cannot do enough for us and are generally so sympathetic and sensitive to the situation. With hindsight, I can entirely endorse the notion that the kindness shown at such times is never forgotten.

Once again, you prove what a great traveller you can be: you are patient and well behaved for the entire trip and when we arrive back home in London again you have been travelling for almost 30 hours.

For the following weeks, I throw myself into helping to arrange the funeral and trying to keep myself busy. You are worried about your grandma and I take you to see her most days. It is a difficult time for you too and I know how much you loved your grandad.

So, sadly, your birthday is overshadowed this year. I have to swallow hard when I open your cards with you and for the first time I see a card signed by just your grandma. To the right of her signature there is a blank space like a hollow sigh, so final and absolute. Bereavement, I suppose, is a sequence of unavoidable moments just like this one.

Feeling at best a little ambivalent towards male authority figures at the moment, I do not entirely welcome the invitation, a few weeks later, from your head teacher. He wants to discuss with me the work that is being done in school by you and the other pupils on the new project. The meeting fills me with apprehension. The deputy head, who was the driving force behind the whole thing, no longer works at the school. Her recent unexpected and rapid departure was indeed puzzling, suggesting to the uninitiated that there was a slightly *political* aspect to it. Your head teacher does not wish to discuss the matter and so we don't. Instead, he brings me up-to-date with what has been happening. Two pupils have dropped out and he no longer has enough staff to cover the extra lessons. You will be able to have your one day of tuition but that will be all. It's possible that some time could be found at the end of the school day, as an 'after-school activity', but that would need to be discussed.

I thought it was all going so well.

I thought the piece in *The Times* would have ignited everybody's interest but it seems I was wrong. Eight months later and it is as good as forgotten. The school has been keen to keep the project fairly quiet and low key, fearing that it would be bombarded by requests from parents or from teachers in other schools, suggesting pupils that would benefit from this sort of teaching. So it has remained a well-kept secret, too well-kept maybe, and then it failed for lack of support. He reminds me that you are still to be taught in exactly the same way but this hardly qualifies as a consolation.

You wanted to make a difference and I thought you were on your way to doing just that.

Quickly changing the subject, he asks me about the work you are doing at the moment and I tell him you have started working on C.S. Lewis's *The Voyage of The Dawn Treader*. In one of the chapters there is a reference to the seven vices and virtues. This seemed to arouse your interest so you spent some lessons working on various ideas around vices and virtues. Then within a matter of weeks this had taken off into whole sessions dedicated to what I could only term ethics. I am actually very excited about this and it's been one of the most fascinating developments so far. You study current news stories and dissect the underlying issues and conflicting moral principles. You are showing yourself to be a highly principled young lady. I explain that this might be the start of another great episode but, unfortunately, he has another meeting starting any moment now.

I return home saddened by what I have learned. Of course I am happy that you are doing so well, that has always been my primary concern. But this particular project was never just about you, it was about sharing something and trying to make something happen for all the other students too. To help find another Secret Garden or two. Now I fear it just looks too much like another wasted opportunity.

I return home in low spirits. When you arrive back from school, I tell your stepmother what transpired at the meeting and that we are sort of working on our own again. She is very sympathetic. Anxious to take my mind off my troubles, she suggests that we arrange a holiday. We could take your grandma too. Give us a few months to sort something out and maybe go away around the time of my birthday. I tell her I think that it's a great idea and ask her if she has anywhere in mind.

She thinks for a moment.

'Venice?'

Before starting your supper, I take you out in your wheelchair for 20 minutes or so. I have no particular purpose or destination in mind, just the idea that we could both do with a change of scene. We make our way over to the park and I sit on the grass next to your wheelchair. A whole sequence of thoughts and ideas connect and disconnect, form and reform and I just want to sit with you like this for a few minutes. I don't need to say anything but the words come eventually.

It has been quite an eventful period for us. Eighteen months ago your mother moved out and last month my father died. Suddenly, this afternoon, for no more than a few moments, this seems to give us some fleeting common ground. It is little beyond the briefest and vaguest psychic connection but it somehow manages to make our own slightly skewed sense of family a little stronger. It is as though we must be careful to protect what remains, as it might be more vulnerable than we think.

With these thoughts in my head, we set off for home as I

am forced to conclude that a season is certainly now passing. Therefore one must surely be about to begin.

You are sixteen years and 119 days old and you appear unusually calm, whilst around you three adults conduct themselves in a state of the greatest agitation.

It is the morning that we are scheduled to make the trip to Dover to collect your GCSE results. The matter seems of such little consequence to you nowadays. I had a chat with you earlier in the day and your only comment was that you were 'no worried'. I don't know if this is a possibly misplaced over-confidence or just a general lack of interest in the subject. Meanwhile your stepmother, your tutor and I run through every possible scenario. You fail both the art and the maths, you fail maths but pass art and so on.

By about 9.30, after about an hour or so of this, we are unable to take the strain of waiting any longer and, nobody is in a fit mental state to drive the 15 miles to Dover. Your tutor calls the school.

Yes.

Yes.

Yes please.

Oh, God.

Really?

Thank you so much!

Then there is a moment that elongates itself so it defies any notion of rational time, on and on it unfurls itself, forever and ever. Then, in wordless confirmation, the expression on your tutor's face tells us all we need to know. You have passed both of your GCSEs.

YOU HAVE TWO GCSEs!

I am so proud of you. And what a great team you proved yourselves to be. The combination of you, your scribe, your tutor and your stepmother working together, has just pulled off

221

something so remarkable, something that so many people would have judged impossible. A young girl with no speech and very little movement has just bagged herself two GCSEs!

Blinking back the tears of relief, gratitude, surprise and sheer wonder, I pick you up out of your wheelchair and we dance around the living room. I know that this is your moment. But just for a couple of minutes, I want all of us to share it.

When the idea of you taking exams was first discussed I did wonder how I would feel if you were to ever succeed. I didn't imagine that it would feel quite like this, not the full depth and intensity of the experience, and I also didn't imagine that the first thing I would think about when I once again drew breath, would be that incident with the yawning.

I must admit that I have not thought about that particular occasion for about 16 years and I can't begin to imagine why its recall should be suddenly prompted today of all days.

It was during your first year sometime. I know it was a disturbed night because it was in the early hours of the morning. It occurred roughly around the time I first became aware that I was generally regarded as deluded or unable to face up to the extent of your problems. Each time I made some positive comment or observation, I was either doubted or treated as though I was in some way mistaken.

On this particular night you were sitting on my lap facing me and I was half watching something on the TV. I remember feeling incredibly tired and I'm sure it was at the end of a particularly gruelling week. I remember I yawned rather extravagantly and then in that typical way that yawning can be so contagious I watched as you did precisely the same. A minute later I did the same thing and again you did too. It seemed such a normal little interlude in a life that, in those desperate hours, usually felt so far removed from any notion of the word. I noticed that you always did this and, during that period, I probably did a lot of yawning! Then it started me thinking and I wondered how this contagious reflex actually worked. If nothing else, it seemed to be strongly suggesting that your eyes were working well enough. Anyway, I remember taking you to the library a day or so later and doing some research.

One of the theories about the contagiousness of yawning involves it being a basic form of imitation and therefore a very fundamental communication skill. Autistic children do not yawn in imitation of others and this might suggest that the impulse to do so demonstrates a level of empathy.

This obviously appealed to me. The idea that you were empathising in some way would obviously be an encouraging sign. Which is probably why I have never told another living soul about it. I just couldn't bear to have that little hope taken away from me, to be told that I was mistaken in some way. It was just something between the two of us and I never mentioned it to anyone, not even your mother, and I had completely forgotten all about it until this morning.

I suppose I could make connections between that moment 16 years ago and this one, to plot a line directly between the two points, but to do so would be to grossly oversimplify the issue. Besides, there isn't time for such indulgences as, within a matter of minutes, we are on our way to Dover to collect your official certificate from the school.

I speak to one of the senior teachers at the school and she is delighted with your results. She says that what you have achieved, particularly in maths, is quite incredible and, in her experience, absolutely unique. She makes a point of congratulating you, and by this point you seem to have cheered up slightly and are giving every indication of enjoying the attention. At one point someone asks me what is next as far as your education is concerned and I confess I have never given it a moment's thought. I have been so completely focused on these exams for such a long time that I have never really considered what we should do thereafter.

I decide to mull it over carefully one day.

But not today.

We return home and I write e-mails, make phone calls and generally make public the news. Meanwhile you continue to demonstrate that commendable lack of interest in your own achievements. When asked how you feel about it all, you simply express the greatest delight that you will never have to do maths again. Or as you rather more succinctly put it:

'happy no maths.'

During the weeks and months immediately following your results, I witness a definite change in people's attitudes towards you. In the past, whenever I have introduced you to people and explained that you are an intelligent young lady, there has so often been a flicker of confusion. Maybe it's the admittedly subjective judgement of a father or perhaps they are simply unable to imagine how such intelligence might manifest itself in a person with your physical problems. Or that your intelligence is simply relative to the intelligence of other people with similar problems. As I am now able to qualify any remark about your cognitive prowess by adding that you have a couple of GCSEs, including one for maths, I am noticing a slight but definite modification in people's reactions. They seem much more at ease with you, more understanding and appreciative.

Beyond all the other benefits, I now realise that, from this point onwards, your GCSEs will serve as a means of quantifying your intelligence, placing it within a more universal criteria in a way that can be more generally understood.

The one curious aspect to all this is that I always imagined that I would feel so vindicated when I was finally able to offer irrefutable evidence of your intelligence. The great day would arrive and I would present that tangible, indisputable, ultimate PROOF that I have been questing after for so many years. I would have thought that on such a day I would feel a sort of righteous elation but I was wrong about this. I simply don't feel like that. It is not something I have actually even thought about.

But today is just a day like any other day, during which I will continue to be quietly overwhelmed by each and every one of your achievements.

You are seventeen years old and for your birthday this year you have chosen to celebrate the occasion with a trip to Moscow. We are accompanied by your stepmother, your grandma and your tutor, who continues to work with you more often nowadays in the capacity of artistic assistant. You were quite adamant about this trip for your birthday and insisted that you wanted to go somewhere different. After some deliberation, you narrowed this down to a choice between Reykjavik, Copenhagen, St Petersburg and Moscow. Eventually you settled on the latter. I was initially quite taken aback by your interest in visiting these places, but I think over the last couple of years, you have developed a real interest in travelling and you rarely express an interest in revisiting a place unless it's particularly special to you.

I think you have fallen for the whole romance of travel and while we usually have to make some concessions to the practical arrangements, like getting your wheelchair on to the plane, etc., I am delighted that you are constantly on the lookout for fresh horizons and new destinations.

However, despite being fascinated by the history of Red Square, the Kremlin and Saint Basil's Cathedral, you are not over-enamoured of the Russian capital. This is partially due to the weather, which is particularly cold and unpleasant during our visit, and the occasionally poor wheelchair access in the older parts of the city. It is once again noticeable that the trip does not inspire any pictures beyond a couple of sketches of Saint Basil's.

It is around this time that your whole approach to painting begins to modify itself. There seems to be a number of different influences at work, some obviously artistic and some a little less tangible. Your stepmother has recently returned from a trip to Japan and, following your study of haiku a couple of years ago, you have always been interested in Japanese art and drawn to the whole idea of simpler, more minimal means of expression. As your stepmother was reading up about Japanese art prior to her trip, she was explaining to you about the different traditions and aesthetics. This seems to have a profound effect on your whole attitude towards your painting. This is not to say that you are painting in a way that resembles Japanese art but simply that you are now incorporating a certain way of thinking in your approach to a picture.

At first it seems as though you are abandoning your drawings before you have completed them. But then gradually it becomes obvious that you are just trying to portray only what you feel to be the essential elements. You are trying to capture in the most simple and beautiful way possible the absolute truth of what you are attempting to depict, and anything beyond this you simply consider to be unnecessary detail.

This new style of painting evolves fairly slowly over a few months. I first notice it in a number of your flower paintings. While the flowers are detailed in your usual representational style, the vase is simply suggested with a line or two. It is all you need to know about the vase but it gives the overall finished pictures a frail and rather serene quality.

What started as no more than a sort of experimentation becomes a very recognisable and definite style. You refer to these pictures as your New Look paintings and as your confidence grows you begin to apply this technique to subjects beyond still lifes. You first attempt portraiture and produce a series of paintings of jazz women (Nina Simone, Bessie Smith, Alice Coltrane and the like). You approach these in a very similar manner and use the same minimalist drawing technique, coupled with a very restricted palette of light browns and greys. The end result is a quite stunning series of pictures that somehow manage to be both deceptively simple and yet highly sophisticated.

They are the works of a true artist.

You spend a lot longer preparing for these pictures than at any point in the past. You produce a number of sketches and in each successive image it can be seen that you are stripping away more and more of your subject so that you are just left with its essential meaning. I'm sure that this manner of working is also physically easier for you; it involves a great deal of mental preparation but the physical effort is reduced somewhat.

What I find most pleasing about these New Look pictures is the fact that you have decided that you want to keep a couple of them. This is something that has happened so rarely, I take it as a positive verdict on your own work. These are pictures that you would like to look at. So your portraits of Billie Holiday and Sarah Vaughan become the only two of your paintings to grace the walls of your room in Canterbury.

Nowadays, whenever I think of you as an artist or as someone who is so desperately keen to explore as much of the world as possible, I realise that these are your own ideas about yourself; your sense of your own identity. They are not ideas being forced upon you by me or by anyone, or being adopted for some sense of the common good. You are now defining yourself in the manner of your own choosing. Your life is being lived on your terms. This is who you are and this is what you are and this, I realise, is just another way of stating that I am slowly accepting the fact that you are rapidly growing up now.

You are seventeen years and 195 days old and you, your tutor and I are back in New Orleans. I promised that one day I would take you back and, having been assured that the French Quarter was more or less untouched by The Storm (as they refer to it in the locality), I thought now would be as good a time as any. We endure a long and difficult journey but the expression on your face the following day as we leave our hotel to explore, makes every minute of it worthwhile. It seems that this is still really one of your special places and, if not the equal of Paris, then perhaps a close second.

Our visit comes at the end of a month or so that has been very interesting from an artistic point of view. Interesting too as once again you proved yourself right and everyone else wrong. Including me, I must reluctantly add. It all started at the end of the summer when we were reviewing your paintings and selecting what you should exhibit in the local autumn exhibitions. There were a couple of beautiful flower paintings that you did at the end of last year that have never been shown. I think that these would be perfect for the exhibition and I remind you that your flower paintings are usually rather popular and fairly likely to sell.

This is true and for the last couple of years, ever since that first exhibition, you have usually made enough money from the sales of paintings around this time of the year to pay for all your Christmas presents.

But this year you have other ideas.

You do not want to exhibit any of your old pictures. This year you insist that you only submit your New Look paintings. I know from experience that when you set your mind on something there is generally no point in reasoning with you but I decide to give it a go anyway. We embark on a conversation that countless artists have had to endure from countless artist's agents, since someone first raised the issue of credibility versus saleability. I am acutely aware that I am simply part of a long and not necessarily noble tradition when I explain that, while I personally think your new work is by far the best you have ever done, it may be better to play it safe and put in a couple of the older flower pictures. But you are absolutely adamant on the matter. You are determined to show the newer work.

Despite my reticence, I have to say that I greatly admire your integrity, although I worry that you might be disappointed if you don't match the sales of previous years. But you want your new work to be seen and this is by far the most important

aspect for you. Besides, you seem confident that the New Look pictures will sell too.

You select the three pictures you want to submit this year. One of which is a recently completed nude. It is actually the first nude you have ever painted. Inspired equally by attending a Modigliani exhibition and looking at a book of Bellocq's photographs of the working girls of old Storyville, it is a very sensitive study. Again I'm not entirely sure that it's suitable for an exhibition of this kind but once again you are utterly determined that it is shown.

The weekend of the exhibition arrives and we submit your work. Your nude raises a few eyebrows but, thankfully, it is selected along with a couple of other examples of your New Look. Before we return on the Sunday, to prepare you for any possible disappointment, I spend an hour or so on the subject of the capriciousness of the bourgeoisie when it comes to appreciating art. As you were so keen to exhibit your new work, I tell you that you must regard this whole experience as a great opportunity to make an artistic statement. Expecting any more than this might be unreasonable.

It is therefore somewhat of a surprise to discover later in the day when we visit the exhibition that *Storyville Nude* has an orange sold sticker on its frame! You seem absolutely delighted about this and I can't blame you. I knew you were so desperately keen to show that picture and you were absolutely right to do so. You have been following very much your own artistic path this year and this must therefore feel like a uniquely personal success for you.

Meanwhile, speaking as one who has just been so recently proved wrong, I should point out that any day that restores a little of one's faith in art and human nature, is generally a spiritually uplifting one.

A few days after the close of the exhibition, the gentleman purchaser comes to our house to collect his painting and hand over the money. He is very keen to meet you. I explain that you are disabled and give him some background on you but as soon as he sees you he introduces himself and informs you that he is an artist too and an art teacher. He explains why he was so impressed with your paintings and from this point onwards, you are simply two artists relating to one another.

Disability is not an issue now.

Art is the only issue.

He tells you that he visits the exhibition every year but this year he was absolutely captivated by your new work. He seems very interested in your new approach and your new ideas and he concludes by affirming that he would have bought every one of your paintings if he could have afforded them. But he eventually settled on the nude because he thought it was so original.

He leaves us after telling you that he will be looking forward to seeing how your ideas develop and what you'll be exhibiting next year.

I will be looking forward to it as well.

Only next time I will make sure I keep quiet and rely entirely on the artist's evidently far better judgement.

As we have both now discovered, faith is a quintessential human virtue, but ultimately we are only questing after that magical moment of fulfilment, confirmation or vindication.

In the meantime we reacquaint ourselves with the French Quarter and, as we stroll around in the sun, I wonder what fabulous new images you are conjuring up in your mind today.

You are eighteen today and this year we are spending the weekend of your birthday in Nice.

Nice is beautiful and I can think of no single place more perfect for a young lady with your particular tastes to celebrate her eighteenth birthday. As might be expected, your initial impressions of the place are those of an artist; you write about the light and the specific shade of blue of the sea. During our stay we visit the Matisse and Chagall museums, both of which you enjoy and I am confident you will find the work a source of further inspiration.

Meanwhile, the date that I have kept filed on some mental calendar for as long as I can remember sneaks up upon us in a French Riviera hotel room as we sleep.

So, here we are then, 18 and today you are now officially an adult. It is another point, another landmark in your life that all but insists I pause and reflect and have lofty thoughts. But as the day staggers clumsily forwards – teetering and reeling under the burden of its own perceived import, I confess the words do not come easily to me today.

I suppose 18 is the point when the relationship between parent and child, between father and daughter, inevitably evolves – by acknowledging the latter's transition into adulthood, one accepts as a direct consequence that the role of the former is being subtly modified. The bonds, of course, remain, but one always senses that there is a slight stepping away required. It is difficult to define or categorise. The love and support remain a constant but perhaps there is a significant reduction in the level of involvement. I don't know how all this will apply to you and me. I imagine that we will at some point find our own *equivalents* as we always do.

But we are in no particular hurry.

With your consent, I'll just keep jamming in much the same way that I have always done and we'll find our way through it all somehow.

A year or so ago when I saw your name on the electoral roll for the first time I began to think about this day and I have often imagined, almost even rehearsed my feelings. Naturally, as might have been expected, the reality of the actual day is entirely different. To be honest with you, it is hard to actually locate my feelings today – they seem to be obscured somewhere behind lapses into overstatement or flippancy.

So I have excused myself the drawing of any great conclusions today. Partly because I realise what a ridiculous conceit such a thing would be. Nothing is being concluded today. This is not a story that ends today – I just thought it might be a suitable point for us to stop and glance over our shoulders.

So, as the day progresses, I allow myself a brief glance or two. One such glance happens around lunchtime. During a brief pause in the celebrations, I push you in your wheelchair through the Sunday street markets of the old town as we take an idle stroll in the approximate direction of the sea. Meanwhile, in the bright sun of midday, on the bleached white pavements, the faded stone buildings with their ancient shutters, on the roads, the sky, the sea and on every available surface, I silently and privately project a series of imagined cine films covering the past 18 years. In the first scene you are small and vulnerable, frail in a way I have almost entirely forgotten; you look frightened, but I can still see so easily that strength of character and personality shining through – sometimes I know I am the only one who can see it. The picture fades and then I can see you confused, angry, frustrated, even tormented, but somehow in the midst of this you still exude such a great sense of inner peace and calm. In the last scene, there is the smile on your face that I know so well. Then, above the smile, I catch sight of a pair of dark eyes that burn like Picasso's with such passion and intelligence.

You have proven yourself time and time again and finally you are defined by what you can do, rather than by what you are unable to do. I concede that this might be considered only a slight shift in emphasis but looking back over your first 18 years, this might well stand out as the greatest victory of all.

In that piece I wrote, or more truthfully overwrote, for the *Independent* about you ten years ago, I said something about mistrusting a happy ending in so far as it blinds us to the unconditional nature of love. Apart from a cringe of recollection periodically, I'd never given the article a second thought but I suppose it seems pertinent today. I think I know what I was getting at. My belief in you has been doubted, questioned and even ridiculed to the extent that there were times when I doubted myself but I don't think I was ever called upon to offer tangible proof of my love for you.

I watched your sleeping face through the glass panel of an incubator exactly 18 years ago today. I was frightened and confused. Just like you. But in that instant there was a connection, like a spark or a star and I felt all the strength and all the patience and all the energy I would ever need to get us through. In other words, it was love at first sight.

There will be challenges and disappointments, but there are in all human lives. There will be anxieties, doubts, there will probably be a few more stupid people in some official capacity or another thrown in our direction and there will be days when any hitherto relatively sane human will just feel like giving up. But we've got this far and we've managed to carve out a little shared history for ourselves – one from which we can draw some strength or some insight in the future. But it has been, and it continues to be, such a great adventure and a great education and I feel so honoured to have been a part of it.

Thank you.

I know that I will continue to derive great strength and hope from you but we both know a season is ending today just as surely as one is now commencing.

Meanwhile I am more than happy to let this day take its own course. Thus it will conclude as it does every day – with me saying your prayers with you as you drift off to sleep. As we do this I will remind you and I will also remind myself that:

ANY DAY IN WHICH THERE IS LOVE IS AN IMPORTANT DAY.
ANY LIFE IN WHICH THERE IS LOVE IS A VALUABLE AND FULFILLED LIFE.

Amen to that, daughter.

Nice, April 27th 2008